EAT NO EVIL

by Roy Masters

Edited by Dorothy Baker

EAT NO EVIL

Published by The Foundation of Human Understanding
Printed in the United States of America

For information, please direct your inquiry to:

The Foundation of Human Understanding
P.O. Box 1009
Grants Pass, OR 97528

Or call toll free: (800) 877-3227

Cover design: Yuri Teshler
Typographer: Ingrid Mauer

Library of Congress Catalog Card Number 87-80407
ISBN 0-933900-12-0

CONTENTS

"Never eat what you like.
Rather, eat what you know
is good for you. Great wisdom
is required here. To eat the
wrong food is to sustain pride
in its supreme folly, so that
pride food poisons not only
the body, but the soul with it."
—Roy Masters

"Many dishes cause many diseases.
A simple diet is best."
—Pliny

Preface

In the classic story "The Wizard of Oz," Dorothy finally discovers—at the very end of her long and dangerous search for a way back to Kansas—that she has always possessed the means to return home. When she learns this truth, she is astonished, dumbstruck, that so mundane and ever-present a thing as her slippers could truly be the means for her finding her heart's desire. Did she really always have, "right under her nose" as it were, what she couldn't obtain from great witches and wizards?

The book "Eat No Evil" will leave you with much the same feeling Dorothy had when the good witch enlightened her—awestruck at the profound and unsuspected meaning and power of so ordinary a phenomenon as eating.

Indeed, food is the most familiar of all man's activities, and the one he suspects least of harboring a great cosmic mystery.

"Eat no Evil" reminds me of a good murder mystery. The super sleuth solves the baffling case by fingering the butler, the familiar and seemingly innocent person least suspected by everyone else. So does author Roy Masters expose man's relationship with his food as the unsuspected, ancient origin of man's problems. He shows exactly how people's hang-ups with food are directly connected to all their other problems.

Roy Masters writes in a way that has become his hallmark—he allows the discerning reader to test and discover for himself the truth of what he says. For if what is written on these pages is true, then there will be a deep down recognition of that truth in the reader.

The average person walks through the supermarket in a semi-dreamlike state, mind floating merrily along with the ever present muzak, cart bumping into those of other entranced shoppers. Unconscious suggestions carefully planted in the mind by television commercials now surface to do their work, controlling the shopper's buying "decisions."

Maybe you're more aware than that. Perhaps you notice that the aisles of cakes, cookies, and sodas that once seemed so tempting to you now are unexciting, even repulsive. In fact, you probably notice as you stroll through the store looking for something decent to eat, that about 95 percent of what is sold as food today is not even fit to eat.

Yet, even if you are aware enough to know that it is important to "eat right," and have read about every diet known to man, you are still less than half way there. To eat right, says Masters, you must get right. And to help you attain to that end, no stone is left unturned in this book. Unlike all other books on diet, this one tells you, not what to eat, but exactly why you have always had problems with food. Once you resolve the underlying traumas, eating right is as easy as . . . pie.

David Kupelian,
Managing Editor
New Dimensions Magazine

Introduction:
Back to the Garden

If you had been born, say, two thousand years ago, you wouldn't need this book. You would be sustaining yourself naturally by eating all the right foods. But alas, you were born in the twentieth century, as if in a cage, a bleak environment of steel and concrete and supermarket-processed food. Need I say more about the devitalized, bran-stripped junk you are eating?

So now it behooves you to thread your way back through the maze of food traumas and conditioning to discover what God intended you to do with the natural bounty he provided.

Food is to the intestines what truth is to the spirit. In both cases, we must keep a clean house. The problem is that a wrong person cannot possibly eat right food. You will see that the primary emphasis is on the spiritual weaknesses that led you into temptation in the first place. Bear in mind that you must *get* right to *eat* right.

Somehow we all know subconsciously that eating the right foods will inhibit the power of our willfulness. Holy men of ancient times fasted because they knew it was the only way to weaken their souls' resistance to God's will and power. Food abuse is the very elixir of pride, and to the present time is sustained by it. The same can be said of sex abuse.

Sex, the lower animal form of love, is awakened by the food sin, and as it is used to sustain the fallen ego, darker perversities appear as temptations to be indulged. From here to eternity, the egos of men ravage the earth, seeking to stroke themselves with pleasure, and they are ruined in the process. The abuse of food and the ravaging of women lead to the ruination of man in everything he does.

If it is true that wrong (forbidden) food was the basis of the ruination of man, and if it is true that the trauma of it awakened the dark side of his nature, then he ought to find empirical evidence of a food/sex connection in his continuing fall from grace. This is to say that if we could somehow be absolved, saved from our fallen state, we could then begin to eat sensible food, food that is good for us and compatible with our bright natures. We could begin to eschew the fancy concoctions that sustain our rebellion against God to be a god, and our gross sensuality should gradually diminish to the point where man, the dying, propagating beast, becomes the regenerating, eternally-living being. The being that God created in His own image.

Perhaps very, very subconsciously we human beings already know that our willful spirit needs food and sex excesses in order to survive as the god over all we survey; and that is why we are unable (unwilling) to give up our exotic ego-animal-sustaining indulgences. Can you see why anything stolen or forbidden is attractive and sexually stimulating? Junk food is a drug and an aphrodisiac.

If we could detect and free ourselves from the original trauma, we would thereby become enabled to make right choices. And if we then chose to eat of the tree of life, sensible, non-ego-reinforcing foods, we would then, once more, be evolving in accordance with our Creator's will, incorporating His identity into ours, forever growing in Him and He in us. His spirit in our soul and His food in our body add up to life eternal.

The meditation exercise will bring you back, through repentance, to the original threshold of obedience to God's plan, a state of innocence in which you will be saved and enabled to make right choices. Before, you were under a compulsion to sin, to eat willfully and wrongly, and to tempt and abuse one another sexually, to mutate and evolve a living hell on earth and in yourselves. Before, even though you had always known about the pitfalls of temptation, and you knew you should resist them, you could do nothing but give in, with full knowledge of the harm you were doing to yourself and to others. Don't you see how the unregenerate ego sees food? It perceives food, as well as all forbidden immoral adventures, as the elixir of true life (that's living, man!), a moral support, a savior and a comforter, through which man polarizes his attitude pridefully to sustain his separation from God to *be* god and purge himself of guilt.

Pride proclaims its rebellion continually in all its sinful relationships. The proud man can have nothing but a wrong relationship with everything, beginning with food and mother and ending in women, alcohol, and drugs.

The first symptom of his fall to original sin that a man notices is a gross thickening of the flesh and the awakening of puzzling and often embarrassing sexual lust. He becomes acutely aware of why mankind's need to clothe itself started with the fig leaf. Having fallen first to the charms of forbidden food, he now falls under the spell of forbidden sexual experiences. They build up his pride to such a pitch that he loses all consciousness of what these sexual experiences are doing to him. He feels like a conquering hero as he goes from one conquest to another, totally unaware that in the process, he is becoming either a cowardly, angry wimp or a violent, woman-violating brute. He feels himself to be the monarch of all he surveys (pollutes), and the king can do no wrong.

The kind of man who hungers for such knowledge pressures a woman unmercifully to give herself up to his use of her. Prideful men feel that the only way they can "complete" themselves is by violating women for their ego gratification. The women who give in to their blandishments do so from a love/hate compulsion and get their revenge by making the men's lives, and those of their children, a misery.

So you see there is no future in food and sex

abuse. It leads only to a downward transcendence of self, to endless pain and perversions. Each gratified perversion "saves" us from the pain of guilt and awakens new, stranger sensations that drive us to seek out kinkier partners for kinkier sex all the way to hell.

It simply does not pay to see food and sex as our "personal savior." To do so sets into motion a devolution process, evidenced by our faulty relationships and the awakening of ever lower desires. It is the way the prideful soul, thinking itself to be good, evolves the body of the beast. The soul, descending through layer on layer of fleshly self as it wakens to his lust, in and beyond the female form, cries out to the original spirit, the essence, the nectar of the serpent, whose appeal to his pride set him on this downward path.

But the father of all prideful beings is the devil himself. If we carry this process to its ultimate conclusion, we will never know God, but we may discover the truth of our having cohabited with Satan in the spirit if we dare to look in the mirror of reality, where we will see that we have been transformed in his image. Having spiritually cohabited with Satan, we have been made over in his imperfectly perfect image, and we are living in the "heaven" of his hell, having become "one" with the father of the netherworld. Here, at the end of our prideful progression, we are free only from the truth.

The ego of the carnal self, desperate to know itself as god, requires woman to add something of her own concoction to the food she offers him, and to allow him the unqualified right to debase and ravage her body. Through the abuse of each other and food, we try to sustain the illusion that we are the lords of the universe, masters of all we survey. The carnal man, to maintain his illusion of supremacy, seeks ever "better" food and "better" women; and all the while, he is altering and degrading their value and purposes through his sick uses of them on his downward journey toward self-destruction.

The more we deny God to be god (always right, never wrong), the more deeply we will involve ourselves with the people, places, pleasures, and intrigues that will surely kill us in the end.

But, luckily for us, we do not have to die to know hell. After sating ourselves on so many of these forbidden delights, we do make contact with that loathsome reality beyond the natural senses. Even though, in our rebellious state, wrong always looks right to us and right, wrong, God has built into our internal guidance system provision for a change of course. Life is a journey up or down in terms of the values beyond the material realm. The soul stands between two dimensions and is allowed enough freedom of choice to "sin" itself into a corner, where it must repent and cry out, "God, what have I done?"

Fortunate are those who see the folly of taking the low road in the first place, those for whom each morning means a fresh commitment to good for goodness' sake; but souls such as these are rare. Most of us fall in line behind the tempter and refuse to wake up until we can no longer avoid seeing the awful truth of our condition and must scream out in pain for deliverance.

Let us take another look at the role food plays in our human dilemma. Have you noticed how the very act of eating makes you more aware of yourself as a sexual being? Do you realize that with every bite you are unconsciously and compulsively killing yourself? Eating isn't the only trauma that affects you this way. It is simply the most basic and apparently natural. But any trauma, whether it is getting caught in a lie, flying into a rage, playing hooky from responsibility—any trauma will awaken in you a troublesome sexual desire.

Now, if there is a sin/sex connection, and if the sin entered through food, then it follows that the very act of eating to keep body and soul alive could be doing double duty by sustaining the sin of pride and sexuality at the same time. Of pride, let me say that it is a sentence of death; and of sex, it is the evidence of the descent of our ego into mortal flesh, where it now perpetuates itself genitally, whereas in a more glorious past, it perpetuated itself by regeneration of the soul.

How then can we separate pride and death from sinning through food? We have to eat. There's no question about that. But how can we eat without sin? How can we overcome pride and guilt without starving ourselves? Might we possibly eat our way back almost to paradise?

Before I answer that question, let's explore the dynamics of the fall more deeply; perhaps the means of salvation will suggest itself to your innermost mind without words.

If I were the devil, wanting to control you by your addiction to sin, I would inject that sin into the manner of your carrying on some natural activity, and I would do it so subtly that you might not become aware that every time you engaged in that "natural" activity, you were being conditioned to sin again. And even if you caught onto the fact that you were being "had" in some way, you still wouldn't know what to do about it. There would appear to be no way out of the dilemma.

If, on the other hand, I were God, I would certainly provide for the possibility of your falling into the devil's trap by devising a punishment for your defection, as well as salvation from punishment, that would appear to be terribly complicated, almost unfathomable, despite its basic simplicity. I would require you to come home to simple reality and drop the heavy burden of pride. To the pure in heart, the way is always clear and uncomplicated. But for the prideful ones, the way is always fraught with complications and questions, an exercise in balancing this consideration against that until each cancels the other out and progress seems impossible.

To carry our inquiry another step further, if we believe in a Creator at all, might we not suppose that He had in mind for us some natural and proper way to handle sexual desire?

And might we not also assume that it was in man's handling of the first sin, the food sin, that he put the reins of his earthly being in Satan's hands and lost his way back to the natural way of relating to anything, especially to his sexuality. By eating the forbidden food, he elected to serve pride and death, and this service is the legacy that has come down to us from generation to generation.

CHAPTER 1

The
Banquet of Life

A compulsion toward food, alcohol, drugs, sex—
or anything at all—has its roots in pride and the terrible willfulness that pride encourages us to express
as our due. *After all, I'm worth it* we say, as we help
ourselves to one after the other of our delicacies or
forbidden delights. Then when we realize we're
hooked, we compound the problem of our addiction by reacting to our evolving symptoms as
though *they* were the problem. Some of us become
quite adept at dramatizing our helplessness against
the awful things that are happening to us. We even
get our friends (fiends, that is) and an occasional do-
gooder to look on us as the poor, unfortunate victim
rather than the author of our own sad plight.

Until we dare to cease our diversionary tactics
and take an honest look at the real cause of our
wrong relationship with the goodies (mostly "bad-
dies," really) of the world, we will be unable to
bring about any meaningful changes in our life.
First we must see that we have created the problem
ourselves through our proud, egotistical willful-

ness. Then we must see that getting mad at the results and doing battle with them only compound the problem.

The frustration and despair that attend our efforts to free ourselves are simply the pitiful cries of our pride as it finds itself sinking in the quicksand of its own creation. It would be better if we simply gave up and did nothing. But, unwisely, we must attack our symptoms with renewed vigor, as though the sheer force of our anger could give us control over the enemy that has enslaved us.

Finally we must submit; before long we are wallowing hopelessly in our sick "pleasures" and seeking solace from the very people and vices that we once regarded as enemies. They *are* still our enemies, of course, but in our hopelessness, we do not see very clearly: in fact, we want neither to see clearly nor to have anything to do with anyone who *does* see clearly. Simply, no matter how much we wish to deny it, we can never completely escape the knowledge that we are not showing ourselves in the best light when we are trapped in a compulsion. Whether flailing about in protest or simply wallowing, we are not a pretty sight. All our hang-ups follow this pattern, whether they are with people, places, things, or whatever.

The ego doesn't take any threat to its supremacy lightly. When it sees that it has been taken captive by a person or a vice, it seeks to turn the tables by consoling itself with whatever it can milk from the once-hated thing. Beware of the "love" that grows out of hatred and resentment! For example, some-

2

thing might upset you, and the tension drives you to light up a cigarette or get something to eat. You see nothing wrong with the way you have re-acted—you have simply found a solution to settle your nerves (although you may be unconscious of the fact that you were doing this).

The cigarette or the tidbit appears as a friend in need, an answer—at the very least, a cover-up—to what ailed you. But many smokes or many morsels later, it becomes apparent that the "solution" or an-swer to your problem has become a problem itself. Feeling betrayed and threatened, we now use anger to avoid seeing the truth, and we attack our smoking or overeating; but our resentment exerts the same power over us that the original tension which drove us to our bad habit for comfort had in the first place. So you see, getting angry at yourself is always self-defeating. That is why you must learn the basic lesson of patience and apply it in all situations.

We get so caught up in the fight against our symp-toms that we fail to see how we are feeding the problem in the first place. Thus, our crusade against our pitiful condition becomes an excellent avoidance mechanism, and we embrace it as a shield against the truth. It's a case of using a lesser, more socially acceptable problem to hide from a greater ego-threatening guilt. It explains why the confirmed alcoholic or "foodaholic" will not give up. He finds a kind of "social security" in his love/hate fixation.

When food becomes a problem, it also becomes an ego challenge. Not only do you enjoy the upset,

3

but the upset so awakens the appetite that you also enjoy eating more. The enemy has changed form. Now, instead of being upset with—say—your mother for having stuffed you to feed her own ego, you do battle with her *spirit* in the food that has become your love/hate hang-up. You love it—and you hate what it does to you. Food has become a way of hating, or getting close to, your mother. Food *is* mother and mother is food. Even after we have escaped her personal power by transferring our affections to others, the obsession with food allows us to remain connected to the *mother presence* that our psyche still craves.

Food becomes the symbolic mother we will continue to need once we have escaped our own mother's tyranny. Some of us, seeing how we have taken on our mother's identity through our compulsion to overeat, grow to hate ourselves as a way of getting back at the mother we hate. We hate ourselves, so we eat to escape our own hatred, and the hatred drives us to eat again—a vicious cycle.

Whenever you respond to cruelty or any challenge whatsoever with resentment, the will of the adversary gets into you, and the violation awakens your sensuous nature. You escape by immersing yourself in your newfound false appetites. You dare not stop struggling, for if you were suddenly to become free of your hang-ups, you would be forced to come face to face with the truth. Your hate has enslaved you to *mother in another form*; all addictions are the result of an emotional transference, and *emotion is the mother of all addictions*.

Mother (or a female-centered father) is usually the source of our pride and ambition; so whenever we encounter frustration, we feel the need to return to her or to the person or vice we have assigned to take her place—be it wife, husband, food, or drugs—for ego support and reassurance. All of our addictions are simply "stand-ins" for the spirit of mother's milk (in terms of her emotional input). Through them, we reconnect to the source of our ego's strength (obstinacy) and pride—little caring that the pride we seek is that which will lead to our downfall.

Let us examine this principle from another angle. Whenever you sin—fall into conflict with God's will—you become incapable of receiving his love, his life within you. The only reminder of his love that is left to you is the pain of your conscience, and when the pain becomes unbearable, you feel obliged to seek a kind of false deliverance in food. In this way you can hang on to your pride and preserve your selfish ego and continue to deny God. Food then serves as the forbidden fruit of Eden. Through mother, it keeps us proud and unaware of our failing. We need whatever corrupted us to sustain us in our corruption.

If food were an original sin, we could use it to set aside God's will in favor of a personal will; but after that we would need it again and again to keep our guilty souls from feeling guilty. Food, like drugs and drink, is used to deny truth and reinforce wrong as right.

The reliance on food as a source of reassurance

and denial is as spiritually genetic as Original Sin, infecting the entire human race and affecting them in the same way. Ambition, frustrated, makes us fall back on food for ego comfort. Even if we are successful, we feel guilty for having succeeded ambitiously, so we "celebrate" with food. Then comes the struggle. We see that we haven't escaped from our compulsions, but have fallen under their spell more deeply.

Let us say, for example, that hate and judgment have made you fall victim to some disease. You will, as a result, by struggling pridefully with the symptoms, give the disease the energy it needs to absorb the rest of your life. You may even enjoy sickness insofar as it enables you in a perverse way to derive a kind of ego security from wallowing in it or struggling pridefully against it. It is not unusual for a person to get so much comfort from his handicap that he becomes afraid to get well! We end up loving what we hate, and when it becomes an intolerable tyrant, we rebel by embracing another evil. We can't seem to get far from evil and the forbidden experiences we need to exist in our pride.

Hostility toward anything at all causes us to fall into a state of pride, in conflict with reality, and awakens in us a need for reassurance from food and sex. We maintain contact with the seductive, reassuring spirit through contact with the bodies and food of women—their spirit and nature—thus taking on their qualities. These contacts are almost impossible for us to give up, because they permit us to exist pridefully and selfishly. They preserve and reinforce our willful existence. Please bear in mind the relationship that exists between mother's presence and food.

A child who will not eat is very often trying to preserve his selfhood against the force of his mother's need to feed her own ego through the child's enjoyment of the food *she has so proudly prepared for him.* If the child refuses to eat, she feels threatened and will often become so *insistent* that she upsets the child, causing him to take on some of her identity with every reluctant mouthful.

Have you ever noticed how attractive food is if it's bad (wrong) for you? *Bad* is "good" for the willful. It helps *It* to exist. Food poisons your relationship with God and paves the way for selfish ambition to exist. The sin self sees food as salvation, a spirit of false comfort. The errant soul is dependent on the forbidden woman/food experience to justify any forbidden lifestyle. The essence of life is simplicity, but the fallen ego loves to complicate things by seeing life as an intricate maze that cannot be adequately covered by any simple value system. The selfish person is therefore free to get lost in the struggle to pick his own pleasant way through the puzzle.

We are all seeking fulfillment through love, but unless we recognize and repent of our unique failing, we will yearn for the wrong spirit through all kinds of wrong experiences. Wrong can become attractive and seem to be fulfilling, but what we wind up with is *"fool*fillment," a fool's paradise. You drink or overeat to deny the truth and make of the lie a *fool*filling reality. This denial of truth becomes

7

another sin, another conflict driving you to need another drink or another piece of cake or candy to forget the guilt of your compulsion, sacrificing all rationality in the process. You drink or eat yourself sick because your ego is addicted to the lie *as the truth* through the ritual of food or drink.

Your problem is what I call the "mouth/sin connection." The lie is a spiritlike nutrient to a corrupted soul, so that you eat to get at the stuff pride is made of. Your mouth is where the spirit of food enters, the doorway to a mystical experience of adventure for the wicked soul. Just let a child find out what he is not supposed to eat, and he will want it. The soul is attracted to what is wrong, because wrong reassures the wrong that is growing up inside us. Thus, we renew our ancient covenant with hell through everything we eat and drink.

Please notice how natural, whole food from the garden rarely satisfies us. We insist that it be spiced and corrupted in accordance with the rituals of the culture we were born into.

Do you see a basic principle at work here? Sin, through the woman/food compulsion, holds the entire human race in its subtle grasp. Once sin has made a home inside you, it must reinforce itself and grow through the very means by which it came into you. You (as It) must sin to survive. But now it is no longer *you* who sin, because now *you* are under a new command. Your mind is no longer your own. It has deserted the command of God to become subject to God's enemy. It is "It" that carnally hungers and thirsts for (self-)righteousness. The dark spirit is taking you over, and gradually it is becoming you.

You yield to your thoughts just as Adam yielded to the intruder's voice in the Garden. It is always there with you to comfort the fallen self, to raise your spirits through images of food and sex. The fallen man is imprinted with the food/woman presence. It is the god of his existence, and he must be in its presence continuously. Unto it does he pray unceasingly.

Tease, when successful, gets inside us and acts as a false self, a false conscience. That false self then is inclined to put its trust in its self-serving deceptions, and *It* in you drives you to do all kinds of ridiculous things for *fool*fillment. It is always ready to deliver you from reality through the lure of forbidden substances. But each forbidden pleasure brings with it the greater pain of conflict, and until you are ready to give up your will to God, that conflict makes you angry, and your anger (denial, really) makes the forbidden pleasure look even more attractive than it did before.

The voice in your mind that keeps urging you to claim your birthright and have your way with the world, formerly the voice of the serpent in the Garden of Eden, keeps striking at the heart of your relationship with God. It bids you to doubt the truth and trust the lie. It beguiles you into forgetting the perfect doubt you should have felt at the first sign of the intrusion into your proper relationship with the Creator. The more guilty you are, the more you must see the wrong as right, and the less patient you are with any other view of the situation. Right becomes boring, even threatening. A problem with food is not just a food problem, but a *metaphysical* one.

Do you see now why the forbidden is so alluring? It is because your soul has been pulled from the ground of its original being and has become little more than the sum of its forbidden experiences.

Without deception, the selfish *you* that you have become would cease to exist. You continue to eat yourself into a gelatinous ball of blubber, because the selfish *you* is not ready to repent and give your life over to God. Every bite reconnects and reassures your fallen self. It reinforces the original misconception, forever presenting death as though it were life, the lie as though it were the glorious truth. I tell you now, as God told Adam in the Garden, *You shall no longer partake of the forbidden fruit, lest ye perish.*

Anger and resentment are our favorite excuses for going to extremes in sensual self-indulgence. The alcoholic will often go so far as to invent a war game with his wife as an excuse to get drunk and/or become embittered with rage. Since resentment is a sin of pride, it also carries with it the pain of conflict, which sees alcohol as a joyful escape. The alcoholic uses his initial upset for one ego-building experience, which, when it leads to conflict, enables him to enjoy a second ego-building experience, his drink, without reservation. If he were only able not to get upset in the first place, drink would not be so attractive to him. No one can really "enjoy" taking an aspirin unless he has a bad headache.

When you were young, you thought—actually, it was not you who did the thinking and dreaming—that you had to fulfill the fantasies of your imagination or else you would somehow be left out, excluded from the banquet of life. Selfish wants seemed so natural that it would surely be a sin against nature to leave them unfulfilled. So whenever you had to face self-denial, you reacted with resentment; and resentment made you want the forbidden object even more. Your world of thought centered around being upset and dreaming lustfully of forbidden pleasures. When your yearning drew opportunities for gratification, you welcomed them with open arms. And so sin made a home in you through that deception.

Whoever overrides your conscience and permits you to sin is not a true friend. He is tempting you with the forbidden fruit only to gain some advantage or to dominate you. Until you are able to see your lovers for what they really are, your perverted concept of freedom will cause you to equate freedom with attachment to them.

You cannot give up your ego supports without ceasing to exist as you are, for to deny yourself the sweet nectar of the forbidden would be ripping the covers off the reality you are still not ready to face. You cannot sincerely give up your various poisons until you are ready to surrender your pride at any cost, even the cost of "life" itself. As long as you live pridefully, reality is death (to the ego); and even though you may give up one vice, you will surely find another to take its place. The grave still waits at the end of the road—you just change vehicles en route.

Of course, there are the diehards, who have chosen their way of death with an unshakable will. Dying of lung cancer, for instance, they insist that life would not be worth living for them if they had to give up their cigarettes. They *love* their cigarettes, like the gourmandizer *loves* his food and the womanizer *loves* his women. "Loving" your addiction or fighting it, you are just a loser until you are ready to throw in your hand and get out of the game.

If you have been able to read this far, chances are you have a stomach for the truth. Chosen from birth, the elect of God, you will find it impossible to resign yourself to a lifelong involvement with the lies and delusions that are so irresistible to everyone else. Of course, you may eat, drink, or have sex too much—and it bothers you. But the difference between you and the others is that you do not like what is happening to you as a result of your overindulgence. You might have stopped a long time ago and given your life to God had you known the way.

Now I ask you to become objective to your thoughts and feelings, for *only* by doing so can you stop being upset with yourself over the problems you have created through your self-indulgence. It is of the utmost importance that you stop being upset with your problems. Remember, the sin came in two installments: first the willful indulgence, then the angry struggle with the results.

Now you must deal with the second part first. It was your proud willfulness that created the problem. When you attack the results with the same proud willfulness, you are simply adding sin to sin. You must go back the way you came, so your first job is to abandon struggle. Don't listen to the part of you that challenges you to get upset in order to prevail. Struggle is what makes egos evolve in conflict with truth. Realize the truth now, and the truth will extinguish struggle as a matter of course. Gone will be the sick fixation to the problem that has kept you from seeing the real core of the matter.

Abandon willful struggle, and the ego will diminish. Face your problem honestly, realize where and how you failed, feel the shame of it—but don't resent it. When you fully realize your powerlessness, when you realize that of yourself you can do nothing, you will see the futility of struggle, and you will find the faith to turn the problem over to a higher power.

CHAPTER 2

The Heartbeat of Your Troubles: Mother's Breast

Many kinds of situations can trigger an all-out food binge on the part of a compulsive overeater, but they all have one common cause: emotion. If we were not so traumatized by past and present resentments, we could not possibly behave in a compulsive way. We would be completely free to make the wise choice in every moment. As it is, though, it seldom occurs to us to question our "right" to resent the people who offend us in some way, even though they may be completely unaware of the effect they are having on us. So we have piled resentment on resentment until it has become our standard answer to the vicissitudes of life.

Before we can hope to make any headway in our "battle of the bulge," we must understand the importance of giving up resentment. With it will go the feelings of emptiness, strange cravings, and restlessness. You must see clearly that resentment is the very heartbeat of all your troubles; and my job in the following pages will be to convince you that this is so.

Surely you have noticed that every time you get upset, you tend to overeat. The reason for this is twofold. On one hand, it provides escape—escape, that is, from the guilt you might feel if you did not allow your emotions to have their way with you. On the other hand, the act of eating, by its very nature, offers an escape fulfillment, a spiritual renewal of "life." All compulsive behavior provides us that escape and renewal, but if we were not resentful, we would have no need to escape or to be "renewed." Resentment rises from ego's failure to find grace in its day-to-day dealings with life. Indeed, resentment *is* the rejection of God's love, creating a need for sensual love.

If we were graced with perfect faith in our Creator, putting no other gods before him, we might find our worldly environment to be puzzling on many occasions, but under no circumstances could it have a traumatic effect on us. All trauma introduces into the unredeemed psyche something of itself, so no matter who or what it is, it becomes part of us. We identify with it love/hatefully and are attracted to it by means of the seed it has planted in us.

Forevermore, unless we find Salvation, the *It* in us will respond to, and grow from, the *It* (the original trauma) that gave birth to it. Before we ever find the opportunity to become God's children, we become, willingly or unwillingly, children of the culture that has claimed us by injecting its values into us.

We are all emotionally attached to something. Something has laid claim to us, and to escape the shame of our bondage, we glorify whatever it is that has claimed us, thus reinforcing its hold over us and establishing our identification with it. Even though we might have hated and feared the original trauma source, the identification with it that came about through our reaction to it—the It in us— needs and "loves" its original corrupter, the mother of what we have become.

Thus, even people and things that we first perceived to be ugly and smelly become beautiful to our eyes and sweet to our nostrils. We are like the goose that identifies as "mother" the first thing it sees after it has pecked its way out of the egg, even though the first thing it sees may happen to be a fox.

For most of us, our fascination with food began at our mother's breast. Along with her milk, we ingested her "love," her ego support, her approval; and as we grew, we learned to play on the ego weakness of mother that prompted her to woo us with special tidbits in return for our approval.

Wittingly or unwittingly, out of pride or out of guilt, mother seduced us with her food offerings. Her culinary creations were her power and her glory, and any disinclination on our part to lick the platter clean posed a terrible threat to her self-esteem. Of course, not all mothers fit this particular scenario in every detail, but it is surely the rare mother who can accept her child's rejection of her "love" offerings, burnt or succulent, with perfect equanimity. Do you see the myriad possibilities that exist in this mother/child/food linkage?

The conformists among us were only too happy to cooperate with mother's bid for approval by pigging out on her various concoctions. To this day we look to food for comfort and reassurance when the going gets rough, and that's why we're in the shape we're in—fat. But how about the rebels who refused to conform to mother's willful ego by stuffing themselves at her table? Have they escaped? No. Many have turned to drink and drugs out of rebellion.

Through mother, you have learned to look to food as a source of security and an escape from the discomfort of stress. Little wonder that whenever you start to get upset, you seek relief in eating and turn to your favorite chef or to your own culinary talent, if you happen to be the cook of the household, for satisfaction. The eater blinds himself to the truth of his craven dependency on food and the provider of food for his sense of well-being; and the cook derives tremendous ego satisfaction from his or her power to turn on and to appease the eater's appetite.

The sex roles vary, of course. It is not always the woman who does the cooking and the corrupting or the man who does the eating and escaping; and today, any attempt to define the essential difference between male and female is condemned as a form of stereotyping and a threat to a person's right to choose his own lifestyle (no matter how unnatural some of those choices appear to the innocent eye).

But the fact remains that until men take over the bearing and suckling of babies, we can trace our preoccupation with food to mother's breast. *Or we can look back still further to the Garden of Eden*, where Eve started the ball rolling with the forbidden fruit. Man, or the "man" in woman, today merely inherits Adam's weakness for woman's food in one form or another.

The eating of food, especially fruit, seems such an innocent activity, and so it must have been in those first days in Eden; but with the eating of the *forbidden* fruit, everything changed. That disobedience to God's express command had to be justified or explained somehow. To achieve this, man had to see himself as separate from his Creator, so pride entered his consciousness and took control.

After reminding his Creator that it was the woman he had been given who initiated the disobedience, Adam began to see Eve in a new way and to become increasingly dependent on her food and sex offerings for his sense of worth, so that in a sense she became his god. Thus, our preoccupation with food and sex is at the very root of our being.

The scientists now say that junk food can cause criminal behavior, but closer scrutiny will show that it is not the chemistry of the food itself that causes aberrant behavior. Rather, it is the excitement induced by the fact of its being forbidden that supports a man's rebellion against authority, against being told what he can or can not do.

Likewise, drink does not make a man mean, but the spirit of the drink, the motivation behind the act of drinking, reinforces man's rebellious and, in social terms, *criminal* identity, even as it helps him to escape from the truth of what he has become through drink. Both food and drink support man in his alienation and rebellion against God. They cast into him the spirit of another dimension until the nature that manifests in man on earth is the same as it is in hell.

Insofar as food and drink have the power to make us feel good, they also have the power to make us willful and mean and to reinforce the hate-proud nature from which the failing self derives the confidence to continue to live as it should not. Whenever the willful, ambitious self experiences frustration and failure, it runs back to the original source of trauma, food and drink, for salvation and renewed confidence. But for man there is always the "morning after" his disobedience to the will of God, and the frustration he feels over his false comforters, food and drink.

Wherever pride is involved, food and drink masquerade as our personal saviors, but the tiny part of awareness that manages to survive in the shadow of pride can cause us to feel guilty for eating at all. We see gross manifestations of this in anorexia [*anorexia nervosa—"pathological fear of weight gain"*] and bulimia [*"the abnormal and constant craving for food"*], but we will deal more fully with these conditions at another time.

Mostly it is fear of facing reality that drives us to stuff ourselves. At other times it is fear of people. After all, if you're bigger than anyone, who would dare to attack you? The man who is bigger and taller and heavier than his associates knows that he is no more likely to be challenged physically than is an elephant, so he equates size with security. He is more afraid of losing his advantage over his fellowmen than he is of a heart attack, so he eats and eats and eats. Bigger is better.

Women, on the other hand, are often so afraid of attracting the wrong kind of attention from men that they eat to make themselves less attractive to the opposite sex. It is their way of handling a deep-seated fear of power. If they have somehow managed to get married in spite of their fearfulness and have been surprised, if not somewhat appalled, by the enormity of their mates' appetites for sex, and the power they wield through it, they will often set about to eat themselves into a repulsive blob in order to dampen their mates' ardor. They, too, use sheer size as a protective shield and escape from fear of their own ugly power.

It is not surprising that so many fat women have been "blessed" with extraordinarily beautiful features. Beauty attracts attention—a beautiful woman can no more slip through her day unnoticed than can a movie star, and very often she just doesn't know how to handle all that attention. So she eats and she eats and she eats to keep from becoming spiritually ugly and wicked. The fatter she gets, the safer she feels.

Returning to the original thought, just everyday failures, like the frustration we feel when our willful, ambitious maneuvering backfires as resentment, will drive us to the false security of food and drink. As long as we respond emotionally, we have no real control over the growing legion of our compulsions, but the fact remains that we can whip all our problems, regardless of whether they stem from simple daily upsets or from more complicated childhood traumas that have driven us to seek mother substitutes, simply by learning how to be guileless, without ego goals, without ambitions, and, hence, without daily resentment and frustration.

Resentment or impatience must *never*, under any circumstances, have the power to turn you on or to motivate you in any way. Resentment awakens feelings of emptiness and insatiable hungers—unreasonable yearnings that, when gratified, breed more of the same.

Being overweight is not a problem in itself. It's the symptom of a problem. Occasionally, of course, the problem is a rare pathological or genetic inheritance, but in most cases we are overweight only because we fail to deal with stress (injustice) properly. We fall prey to the *respond-and-stuff-yourself* compulsion.

You know that when you become emotionally upset, you get nervous and weak, and before you know it, you feel compelled to eat. But you may not realize that eating is not just a pleasurable experience. It is also a hypnotic fix just like any other escape mechanism; so when you have learned to understand your compulsion to eat, you will also understand the compulsion to smoke, drink, take drugs, or whatever else it is that people do to escape facing reality. Is it possible your mother upset you into eating her peace offering?

You actually experience two hypnotic fixations with every sin. The first occurs when you become upset and fail. You then come under the compulsion to do or say or simply think something that you

22

would be ashamed of under normal conditions. So, sure enough, when the emotional smoke clears, you *are* ashamed of yourself, and your next compulsion is to run from the pain and embarrassment, to escape the awful truth of what has happened to you. In other words, hypnotic fix #1 numbs your awareness, so that you fail to feel the pain of something gone wrong; and this sets you up to need hypnotic reaction #2, the escape into forgetfulness through pleasure.

Neither pain nor pleasure is hypnotic by nature, but when pain reminds us of our failure and pleasure makes us forget that failure, we are dealing with hypnotic forces. Reaction #2 is simply a means of rejecting reality a second time in order to escape the guilty awareness of what went wrong the first time it was denied. It always consists of some form of ego indulgence, usually pleasurable—first, food, and later, sex. But it often expresses itself in another round of resentment.

A person can easily become addicted to being angry all the time in order to feel secure, but this is an illusory and temporary security, and sooner or later he will need relief in the form of distractions from the pain of resenting and judging all the time. And that is where thought of food reemerges. Food can corrupt and change us to need food. One of the peculiarities of hate is that it produces in us a wrong kind of need which we see as love—in this case, for food. If you hate it, you're going to love it; and we allow ourselves to be ruled by that love.

Food sets us free from conscience, and keeps us

free from conscience, but enslaved to the spirit of food—a state we call love.

Food can induce, posthypnotically, an altered state of consciousness that assures you all is well because you feel so good. Surrendering to the source of love puts your soul asleep to the knowledge of your sins. It is like an evil salvation for the preservation of your ego, and while you bask in the comfort of it, the next sin you must escape from through "love" takes root and grows.

Eventually you must realize that conflict, guilt, anxiety, and feelings of aloneness and uncertainty are simply the whimperings of a tormented conscience, and there are only two ways to handle a bad case of conscience. One is to face the truth, admit your error, take your licks, and repent. The other is the egotistical way of denial. In this case, everything you grab onto in your struggle to escape draws you into another presence.

It is not always the food, drink, dope, sex, or whatever, that reduces you to a state of utter dependency, but rather, it is the spirit of the lie that lures you into a false sense of self-worth with rebellion objects of consolation. The fix distracts you from your shame, while the sin reinforces the rebel spirit of false hope and pride.

The compulsive relationship you have with the food or drug is one step removed from the source (pride, anger, fear) through posthypnotic suggestion. Once the hypnotist gains control of the subject, he can transfer his authority to anything he chooses, even inanimate objects, and, thus, maintain his control over the subject even when he is not physically present. Even though the hypnotist may die, his spirit will live on through the subject's reactions to his firmly planted suggestions.

When a husband or wife dies, you will often see the bereaved one clinging to nostalgic objects, photos, clothing, and the like, to seek solace for feelings of loneliness and despair. Through a kind of hypnotic transference, these objects acquire the power to connect the soul to the reassuring presence of the departed spirit. Any encounter with persons, places, or things, badly met, is traumatic; and it is trauma that charges these persons and things with a special presence and power to control us through its suggestions. So it is no coincidence that every time you suffer frustration, you stuff yourself with food. Food represents the consolation of a mother.

Before you can overcome your addictions, your soul must be released from the grip of sin. So look into your mind. Observe your craving and observe your excuses. See how they are connected with the past, and see, also, how you are reinforcing them by your resentments in the present. By not running away, by not escaping into the arms of comfort, you will feel old pains, anxieties, and guilts coming back to be resolved in a new way. You will experience flashbacks. You will receive insights as to how food and mother figure in your particular problem.

Here is one classic scenario: by resisting your impulse to eat, you displease mother; and since you need her approval for your existence and she needs to live her life through you, you will feel guilty for not indulging in her pleasures. Good! Hold it right there. Feel guilty. Don't let mother take your guilt away. If she does, she will become your lord and savior; you *and your sick ego* will have more and more actual guilt for being less and less "guilty," if you see what I mean.

Because it takes you out of the present moment and delivers you into the spirit of corruption, food gives your ego the illusion of salvation. But what it does, in fact, is reinforce the deeply hypnotic relationship you already have with the spirit of corruption through the corrupter who originally seduced you. So stop looking at your comforts and pleasures as the good life; the truth is, as you have indulged in them, you have simply been sinking deeper into a hypnotic trance.

In case you are saying to yourself "I am not asleep," let me warn you. A trance is not a state of sleep. It is an altered state of consciousness under the control of a person, place, or thing to which you are devoted—so devoted that you feel you cannot live without it; but believe me, you can. If you will just learn to be calm and patient, you can resolve all your compulsions. First you must give up resentment. It is killing you.

CHAPTER 3

Forbidden Fruits:
Life's Elixir

Nothing is harder to do than to make an alcoholic face the fact that he has a drinking problem or to convince a fat person that he has a problem with food. Now, it is common knowledge that alcohol and eating are not really causes; they are the symptoms of something much deeper.

Giving up eating or drinking is painful, because doing so will expose the underlying cause that threatens the ego—some past sin, shame, or failure the ego is denying. It is possible not only to drink to forget the guilt of drinking or the disgusting things done in a drunken fit, but also to eat to forget the sins that slip through our gluttony.

Surely if eating and drinking are a denial of our faults (the same thing as denying the saving grace of truth), just as surely, then, do we set ourselves up to commit more sins to deny. And if that is true, then we shall just as surely be committed to the only means we know to deny the truth of those mistakes: eating to forget the guilt of eating, drinking to forget the guilt of drinking; this is the poison of forgetfulness.

If it is possible for an alcoholic to drink to deny the truth, then that poison, which denies reality (the very truth which has the power to redeem him from the past sin), sets him up for the next trauma. Gluttony and drink, then, represent rebellion and stubborn pride.

What I am trying to say is that alcohol can be a second-stage denial of something gone wrong further back and forgotten. The first problem, the first sin, did not originate through drink, but stubborn sinning led to drinking as a potent means of denying the truth of the original sin. Without doubt, alcoholism is connected to an original trauma, and I am implying that that trauma was, and still is, food.

All cultures have the same problem with food; and like alcoholics, few realize it, because cultural food is the worst kind of drug. Our problem with food has led to every problem we have ever had and ever will have; it has led also to the use and abuse of ever stronger means of denial for dealing with evolving guilts and problems.

Eating wrongly has been a problem of man ever since Adam ate the forbidden fruit and fell from grace. Why *did* he eat of the forbidden fruit? Because it symbolized rebellion. Adam believed he could become something, acquire something, attain to something forbidden—independence—through that eating experience. So, if long ago that fruit (forbidden food) was sin, it introduced sin (failing) and guilt.

It follows now that if such food can set aside conscience to allow wrong to occur in the first place, then food can be used again to deny that wrong in the second place. The guilt of eating can be assuaged by eating more forbidden food—just as drinking can be used to forget the guilt of drinking. Food, in the same way as drink, is a soul drug that makes reality a lie and a lie—the dream—a reality.

In order to go on rebelling, being prideful, denying reality, we need food to keep us in a stupor, just as the alcoholic craves drink. Sin is also addictive. Once you partake of food to free you to sin, you cannot stop partaking of sin. Sin itself is compulsive and becomes your whole ego life; food and drink make the lie life bearable, believable, and livable.

For most people food is central to life; drink connects to the source of false life. Of course, a life of sin is not limited to the food and drink experience, but this author claims that the human tragedy began with food. This author also claims that we hide a multitude of sins behind gourmet cooking—and because we do, we keep adding error to error and somehow, as will be explained, all the suffering and tragedy, all the illnesses, the mental problems, the emotional problems, the personal marriage dilemmas, and all the physical sicknesses dovetail into original transgression.

A Jewish mother puts something of herself into her food that creates a Jewish man. Likewise, pasta produces Italians in the image of their culture (through mother). Somehow, food as mother prepares it *suggests* into existence the cultural man. Through a nice dish of "people" rump steak, a mama cannibal builds a fine, upstanding cannibal character, if you see what I mean. Perhaps you get the point: In a sense, we are what we eat.

We derive some kind of ego hope, some kind of lying suggestion, that reinforces what we have been made into through mother's "loving" hand—everything that has gone wrong with us seems to be made right through food.

Food is very attractive when we are depressed, just as alcohol is attractive to an alcoholic when he is miserable with despair and anxiety. So, whenever we want a lift, a false hope, we resort to food, drink, and drugs. But I want you to see where the problem really lies. Something more has gone wrong with us through food, just as something more goes wrong with alcoholics through alcohol that makes them go back to alcohol to make things right. Of course, everything becomes worse under cover of our "happy" stupor—it just sets the stage for the next tragedy. And how do we deal with that? More food, more drink.

Mysteriously, food, which allowed evil to enter our lives, helps evil by denying the truth that something is wrong. A stubborn, rebellious ego is involved here. Sin (through food) has this kind of power over your mind. Sin sets aside your conscience to free you, permit you, to do the wrong in the first place and then again sets aside your conscience about what you have done wrong in the second place. And that's how we get hung up with it all. Food consoles.

Food is a consoling (and condescending) mother.

It tells us that all is well with us and our world. Food lies. And the ego has a love affair not so much with food as with that which lies beyond evil: deceit. So it's obvious one cannot help those who are not willing to face the truth. Their answer will always be to embrace the spirit—their lord and savior—at the sacrificial altar of food and drink. As long as you are stubborn, not willing to face the truth, I cannot get you past this place. There's no point in your reading any further.

It is all a matter of pride. Pride and all the problems that come from being prideful (denying reality through food and drink) will be perpetuated through food and drink. You won't be able to see where all your problems are coming from; you will blame others for your troubles. You must see that your attraction and fixation to, and your fascination with, drink is simply a matter of the falsely-based allegiance of pride to the sustaining evil.

Food and drink nurture pride, and as long as you are willful, you have no other choice but to eat and drink yourself to death (even though you may see it as life). Food and drink reinforce the stubbornness of pride, renew the rebellious nature, and give it the false hope of its lie source. That lie through food is the hope of all prideful beings everywhere. There is nothing anyone can do for your incorrigible, egotistical being—you are simply stuck with your poisons and all the associated diseases, tragedies, emotional miseries, and intrigues.

Food, then, is the first of all traumas, giving rise to love and hate. But there is something special about the shock of trauma that you should know, which is that it not only makes you forget, it changes you so completely that whatever is obnoxious to you before the emotional impact of a traumatic experience becomes exciting and attractive after your trauma. Don't let me traumatize you now by citing a revolting example, but sufficiently traumatized (injured), a person can be made to enjoy eating his own feces or even drinking blood, for that matter.

What was repulsive *before the upset* (trauma) with it becomes attractive after you have been stricken *by* it. What do you suppose makes the wrong kind of food always attractive, and the right kind boring and unattractive? Why do you suppose that you are mated to the wrong type of man or woman? The truth of the matter is that you are attracted to the vehicle of the reassuring lie throughout the entire spectrum of life's experience.

Wrong is attractive because your whole sin/ego existence has come down to revolve around it. The moment a child finds out what he or she is not supposed to do, that is the thing he or she will want to do. It becomes exciting, and wrong excites feelings of ego life. The minute children find out what junk food is, junk is the food they demand. Studies have shown that character can be modified through the eating of forbidden food and that criminal behavior can be triggered by junk food. Now, how on earth can sugar or chemistry create criminal behavior—change a person into a thief or a murderer? Of course, logic dictates that it cannot.

It's the spirit that enters *through* the experience, the trauma of the forbidden; that is what does the harm and causes personality change. Pride, then, is dependent upon forbidden experiences—dependent on the spirit of sin to feel secure in its wickedness. Pride is dependent on the excitement of sinning for evolving a false sense of identity—nurtured by repeated contacts with its traumatic source and cause—that is to say, crossing over the forbidden zone, where its life is, and escaping reality.

Through a forbidden experience or trauma, something goes wrong and overthrows our true self to grow up in its place—the unholy in the place of the holy, perpetually renewing itself through wallowing in the sin of food and drink.

We simply cannot see anything wrong with drugs or sexual immorality, stealing, murder, or rape or recognize that they resulted from our having been violated. Think of it—we can delight in being raped or violated, because it means we are in contact with the (evil) god of our origination! Trauma is renewal, *re-creation*. Food and drink are portals through which a re-creation spirit enters and evolves. Once sin has been experienced, sin then seems the natural state. One sees nothing wrong with stealing, once one has been violated or tempted to steal.

To a vampire, blood seems the natural food. Once he has been transformed from man to zombie and become a vampire, another's blood is not only the vampire's whole life, but indulging also serves as a means of forgetting *what he is and also what he might have been*, had he seen by the light of reality. Blood, then, is a means of forgetting shame, denying truth in order to go on being what he has become through the blood. The vampire's life comes from corrupting, and the victim's life comes from being corrupted and being transformed into zombie and then, perhaps, vampire. In real life some of us remain zombies while others go on to become "mothers," manipulating food, drink, drugs—"consuming" us as we eat and drink.

In this light, sin (for victims) can be seen as two things at once. First it is denial or forgetfulness, and at the same time it is the renewal of the implanted ego spirit of pride. Through food you are transformed, and you also forget what grew inside and changed you; you grow the sin self as though it were the true self. You forget that what you are is wrong; and you remind yourself that *error* and the deviant, sickening you, is right. And through food, wrong is denied to the death. Food, then, is a drug.

It should go without saying that food doesn't need to be a drug. Hay is not a drug for horses or cows or sheep. It was by means of a certain food, the original fruit in the garden, that God made his will known. Such food allowed man to choose to obey God or to become his own alien(-*ated*) god. Ever since, man has striven to maintain the illusion of godliness through food. He has used food to deny God in order to become God. Through food we are all being guided by the dark spirit to a "heavenly" hell on earth. Hence—all suffering and tragedy.

Now let me say all this again in a different way. One does not necessarily have to be overweight to have problems with food or to have all life's problems based on eating. One can be perfectly trim and muscular and *apparently* healthy and yet have many serious problems based on food. You need not have an obvious problem with food, as an overweight person does. Remember that food is a powerful dream potion. That's why I implore you to read on and discover yourself in these words.

Problems arising from food are terribly subtle, because eating, in the sense of right and wrong, is natural. Food is involved in our normal ego survival as well as our natural existence; it seems a part of our complete self, our culture, which we rarely question, because the cultural man (the corrupted man) is who we are. Thus, for both usual and unusual reasons, we rarely suspect that something is going wrong with every mouthful, even though we may be trim and healthy. Does it have to come to gluttony and overweight and finally disease for us to see that we have a problem with food? Do we have to bring about family problems even to suspect that we might have a problem with drinking?

Be thoughtful. Pause and ponder this matter. Food is the cause farthest back in time. Drink and sex problems, and so on, which are also causes, are closer and must be dealt with first!

The question I want to pose to you is this: Is it possible to have an identity other than your own, one laid on you by your culture—specifically, by food and mother? Who might you be, were you not brought up on spaghetti, tacos, or matzo ball soup? What kind of person might you have been if you had not been subject to the influence of a Jewish mother? You might have been a cannibal with a cannibal mama—or you might have been a child of God. Whatever you would have become through other cultures, other mothers, other suggestions, other cultural food, you would not be what God made you, and there is the rub—the anxiety and the conflict.

Food has well-known hypnotic and posthypnotic powers. Initiations into various cults throughout the world and subcultures within cultures involve dietetic rituals. Change the food, and you can change the man and sustain him in the altered state. You can suggest what this new man should be, and this new man will depend on ritual eating to remind him that he is indeed that person and to keep his corrupted ego from becoming insecure (shaken by the light of truth). It is the purpose of this text to help you to find and separate from the subtle, seductive mind control techniques and factors that are transmitted through food.

One of the famous Jackson Brothers' singing group gave our organization a Bengal tiger. The newspapers picked up on the story, saying it was no "ordinary" tiger—it was a *Jermaine Jackson* tiger. The effect of this story in the press triggered an immediate and unhealthy interest in our tiger. It was as though something of value—something of Jermaine Jackson—were being transmitted through the tiger, which eager young petting hands needed to experience. The hands of a healer can likewise transmit a curse (in the guise of a blessing).

What I am saying is that if the tiger can transmit something of Jermaine Jackson that all the kids want to get their hands on, to feel the experience, to renew the Jermaine Jackson identity through the tiger, then how much more can mother's food convey the same type of thing without anyone's suspecting harm? If false love and reassurance can be transmitted through a tiger—Jermaine Jackson "love," Jermaine Jackson approval—and if just touching the tiger renews the spirit of the children (the Jermaine Jackson spirit of the children), then how much more can food translate the reassuring will and spirit of mother? Perhaps this illustrates my point; *mother-based people are lovers of food and drink.*

I will prove that food is mother's "love." It represents mother's false love even when mother isn't there, just as the tiger transmits whatever Jermaine Jackson is, even when he isn't there. I've made the point about the tiger to show you how much food can reinforce the mother-transmitted Jewish, Italian, Russian, or other cultural identity; and at this point you should see that women and food are connected—mother and food being translated to wife and food. And food represents mother's love— woman approval—the spirit and the will of mother operating as your own life and will.

Not only does food represent mother—mother's approval, mother's comfort, and mother's presence—but also her spirit. The bottom line, for men at least, is that reinforcement of the ego self is of the consoling spirit of sin—women and food leading to drink and heavier truth-denying vices. The self we are reinforcing is an ego-spirit self, the one created by mother's food. And so, through the wrong type of food and the wrong kind of women, we go on reinforcing the evil inside as right. And that's why everything in our life is insane, backward, and death-centered.

Remember, I said that whatever was obnoxious before the trauma becomes attractive after it. Well, there is another thing you should know about that shock experience (sin), which is that the victim (sinner) becomes increasingly sensitive to everything in the surrounding scene connected with the event. Food by the hand of an "understanding" woman, then, incorporates woman herself and, of course, in a more subtle respect, the *will and way* of that woman.

Women are the keepers of the lie all aspiring egomaniacs need. That's why we select (and serve) wrong food and pick wrong women—cultural food and cultural women who are possessed of the spirit that re-created us egotistically in the first place. And the woman-corrupted *male ego* craves and demands a woman's reinforcing presence. We are always being drawn back to the scene of the crime to reexperience lower and lower sin sensation— now as original love from the original (evil) god.

To illustrate the point in a different way, in a negative way: if you find yourself becoming afraid of everything in life, it is because of the trauma of resentment. Resentment is judgment, and judgment is the other sin of pride, a trauma. Trauma renders you sensitive to, and afraid of, everything in your environment, beginning with the hate object. And you become more and more afraid of everything through resentment.

If you resent your mother or your father, your ego then immediately becomes addicted—*sensitized*—to being resentful but, at the same time, hypersensitive and obedient to the tempter. Resentment must be experienced again and again, for through the sin of resentment comes excitement, the very substance of your ego identity, which came in through that first resentment.

Through resentment, the sin self—the proud and egotistical self—entered; and it makes you go on being resentful in order to sustain itself in you. You need (in other words, *love*) to hate the parenting hate object. But that resentment, which separates you from God's love, makes you subject and sensitive to, and needful of, everything around you. Immediately you compensate with the objects of the scene surrounding the sin, and that is false love.

If you resent your mother or father, pretty soon you resent everybody, and pretty soon you resent everything connected with those you resent. You fall from God's sustaining love, become sensitive to women's clothes or a woman's voice, and begin to compensate with her damaging love. Your sense of direction depends on being close; and yet what you need, when you get it, kills you. Though you may realize it, there's not a damn thing you can do except hate her; and that only makes her more attractive and powerful!

In essence, trauma has both a positive and a negative side, attractive and repulsive. If the trauma begins with seduction, flattery, food, sex, or wine, it can draw you with its vicious, magnetic lovers. You might like to go on to your local bar, for instance. Everything about the bar scene becomes more and more attractive to you—the glistening glasses, the odor of liquor, the music, the noise, the little cocktail trappings.

You feel more and more secure and at home with a "good" woman, because it is there where you draw the elixir to your ego. You are drawn deeper into the wrong environments to reinforce your faulty self. But when the sin partner is revealed as the betrayer, love becomes negatively charged—as it does through resentment—and the same thing happens but in reverse. Everything can become repellent, negatively charged. You could become dependent on the hate object: your wife, your work, your pusher.

In this way do you become positively affected by a woman and also repulsed by her, driven off to the arms of another lover (betrayer-to-be). You can be turned off by anything you once "loved" as you discover it has betrayed you. Discovery of the truth is one of the basic causes of resentment. "Love," being a violating and violent deception, and deception being discovered for what it is, leads to betrayal and, inexorably, to resentment. As a result, the person you were once attracted to and were sensitized by, drawn to, and involved with, now affects you in an exactly opposite way and becomes repulsive to you. Or you can become terrified by your beloved, yet remain strangely needful of that same person's love.

You can need love and yet be afraid of what it does to you to the point where you are unable to approach the object of former love and turn now to another lover and potential betrayer. In the beginning, one never consciously sees the betrayal; your ego sees only the understanding lover. Indeed, some never, ever see the betrayer, for their stubborn egos are dedicated to the death to sin.

Because of her love and food offerings, all men are emotionally involved with women, affected by their enticements—by the lying lips, words, form, and, last but not least, the woman's god (the ancient Demon). Men are immensely attracted or repulsed by women, but, either way, increasingly sensitive to the woman's form of being. You can be terrified, drawn magnetically, yet think compulsion is true love for—and from—the true self, with all the wrong experiences with all the wrong types in all the wrong places.

In short, we become increasingly sensitive, whether it be the sensitivity of repulsion or the sensitivity of rebellion/attraction; the self born of love and hate evolves amidst objects—people, places, and things connected with the scene of the original traumatic intrigue. This explains why men are attracted to women, so affected by them, so sensitive to their presence, and so easily manipulated by them. It can explain, perhaps, why men are outraged by them to the point of bringing on

41

themselves all the problems of rejection—lust, impotence, and fear to the point of terror or desperate violence in order to free themselves.

The dilemma of being attracted to women, on one hand, and being hateful and afraid of them, on the other, is all connected with food, because through Original Sin, pride came into being through eating the forbidden fruit. By the hand of woman, everything connected with, and surrounding, that scene, the food-eating experience, which mostly comprised the presence of woman and her spirit, her consoling foods, enters into the total effect on our psyche and mind and body.

As a man, you may first be attracted to a woman who is greatly like your mother. The transfer of power from the dying queen *Mother Superior* is made through sexual sin. You don't even see, let alone understand, why you were drawn to the familiar spirit of corruption. The key here is that you may not notice the sin, because the sin contact—sex—seems to fulfill a natural need; yet you know that it (sin sex) isn't natural, because of the way it addicts and creates terrible fear and confusion. But in time you may suspect something wrong with your relationship. There must come a time when every man realizes this, then rejects it with booze or drugs and a new love.

While sex is not necessarily sin, even as food is not necessarily sin, the ego needs a forbidden type of extramarital sex, because no other type of sex will reinforce or console the sin self. The self that entered through food cannot tolerate the right kind of *any* thing. Hence, sex outside marriage, or perverted, kinky, unnatural sex is always more and more exciting.

Remember the rule for the ego: Nothing can be experienced in a natural way; everything must be perverted to allow the spirit of pride to enter and stand unholy in the temple of the Holy.

You are addicted, beginning with food and going on to sex and alcohol and all the other cultural "know-nos." You're addicted to love/hate objects; but in either case, in essence, the root is death-centered existence, a fascination with trauma, sin, evil. And the only symptoms may be a troubling anxiety, fear, and tragedy, and you see lots of things going wrong with your life, but you won't know where the hell it's all coming from. You *won't* see because of your habit of *not* seeing, as the result of your love of experiences, your love affair with sick friends, food, and drink. They all set you up for the next mistake. Their "love" sets you up and makes you forget that you are making a mistake and their love *is* the next madness. They are the *mothers* of your existing.

Your pride has grown through worldly delights; the only self you know and want to know is nurtured through deeper indulgence and involvements. The wrong in you grows as the projection of wrong in them; and the hunger grows and is never satisfied—it is the will and purpose of hell on earth. Food is central to the surrounding scene, and the surrounding scene is what affects us and creates another chain of compelling sins. Have you wondered why you are sensitive to everything lately? Now, you know.

In sum, men are attracted to the environment that begat them—the wrong woman, the wrong food, the lying lips and words, and the lying spirit. All are used to *escape* and to reinforce a construct— the fallen alien self—out of the ruins of a paradisaical self. Men are attracted to that scene, and women are obliged, through the sheer demand of man's need, to *be* that scene. And guileful women know full well that the way to a man's heart is through his stomach.

Your increasing sensitivity to stress, your failure to cope, is connected with (the love of) the escape into food, into women, and into the lying spirit wherein lie your foolish hopes and dreams. And so ends your existence on this accursed earth.

CHAPTER 4

The Way to
a Man's Heart:
The Deadly Nectar

Who was it who said that the best way to a man's heart is through his stomach? What a revealing statement that is! For a man's soul is connected to a woman's will through his belly and his genitals—in that order! What mother originates, wife completes. An "ego*testicle*" fate is sealed at birth.

Observe in every culture the common denominator of manipulation—spicy food and women. The mother-centered male craves ego-reassuring food and the form, woman, identified with nourishment of his soul.

The original sin for man was, and still is, ambition—that is to say, the desire for the exalted state such as God has. Before Paradise was lost, man was himself; his will embraced divine will, and the divine love was his existence. Adam's self had no will or existence apart from the Creator self. But through willfulness, doubt, rebellion, disobedience, and the desire to be more, came separation and the transference of allegiance to the woman's will and the selfish life of her love. And so the history of abject human misery began to be written.

From the very first denial, choosing deteriorated into a compulsive, slavish process of denial. The yearning for female love, and love fulfilled *to this day* remain a denial and the pride of life. The re-created one's thoughts and desire are toward *his* cause. Fallen man is obsessed with his re-creator. The love of women seems to man identical with completion—with evolution of his ego.

In choosing the independent path to self and glory, man cannot—often will not—stop embracing the dark spirit of false love, the reinforcing origin of his selfish existing. Man is the effect of a trauma, a lie cause subtly centered within the female form, and the evolution of his ego beast continues to depend upon the traumatic rituals of deceptive love and spiced food.

The *Bible* records that the first man's (outer) eyes were opened through partaking of the forbidden drug of (mind-expanding) fruit. Coincidentally, the trauma of sin closed the inner eye of spiritual perception and reception. Once the inner eye (life from enlightened reason) was closed, the fallen ego began to adapt into its evolving animal self by way of perpetual trauma, scenes of food, women, the deceitful word, and woman's spirit beyond the spoken word.

Excitement, traumatizing and transforming the soul, addicts it to the motivation of its source, a false life emanating from the excitement of the trauma scene and source, which is the woman, the spoken word, the food, and the spirit. "Naughty" woman is the core, the ground, of the male being.

Later on I want to go over the four factors of conditioning—the (forbidden) food, the woman, the spoken word, and the lying spirit of the female.

Like a gosling that is imprinted by, and takes to be mother, the first thing it sees after emerging from the egg, so is man fixated to and imprinted (impregnated) by the woman who originally opened his eyes to *her* presence, her will, to take his identity and purpose from her word through her perverted (cultural) food.

However, before we delve into that subject, let us take a brief look at the psychodynamics of natural foods versus adulterated foods and work back from there. Later we will ponder the disease-producing factors of altered food. Can you see that natural food can hardly corrupt the will, except it itself be specifically forbidden or used in a wrong way, which is to say, the use of "good" health food to effect the salvation of the person from the sin of "wrong" food? When food is used to save from sin, it is another sin. Christ saves, food cannot. Food introduces sin (disobedience through doubt), but right food cannot save from the sin of wrong food. Most people foolishly think it can and put their faith into health fads, adding sin to sin.

The Creator has prepared a natural table before all his creatures. So, if it is true that man has fallen through a forbidden experience with food, the question arises, how does he return to his paradise state? The answer is through eating right, but *through repentance of pride first.*

Living food is everything a creature needs. Horses, cows, and sheep change "unbalanced" diets of straw into healthy muscle tissue, teeth, blood, and bones. Spiders eat flies, koala bear change "unbalanced" eucalyptus leaves into bone, hair, blood, and flesh—and so on.

What do you think would happen if you fed a diet of cooked straw to a horse—or eucalyptus "strudel" to a koala bear? You don't have to be a scientific genius to answer that; they would surely sicken, prematurely age, and expire before their time. The valiant veterinarian battling for his honor and their lives could do very little.

Diet keeps all creatures in their appointed ecological place. Diet is life, and it is also their identity. With diet we restore the animal to its former health; but with man, food cannot undo entirely the sin of what food wrought. Through rebellion, food caused sin to enter; food (or drugs) cannot cure sin. On the contrary, the way we relate to food reinforces the sin of pride that came through food. We crave the wrong kind of food, and when it is health food, it is simply pride trying to make itself better.

What if, for example, the docile, grass-eating sheep adapted to digesting meat? Were it possible for the creature to cross the boundary of herbivore to carnivore, the life of the creature would change. Meat, being the stress/need instrument of change, would then alter the identity and character from a peace-loving to a flesh-tearing creature.

Assume, for argument's sake, it were possible for a sheep to change its nature. Could it then eat grass?

No, it would need its old gentle nature back to do that.

While man happens to be omnivorous, he cannot eat without sin; which is to say, without enlightenment, the curse continues to flow through the food/woman experience to build the ego beast in him that sin gave birth to. Cultural food maketh the cultural man, be he cannibal or Hindu or whatever. And bear in mind that the corruption of trauma is a kind of birth. What corruption changes, corruption is needed to sustain.

Could it be that mankind, through a choice (which animals do not have), has crossed over to the forbidden zone, changed and adapted to a cultural existence revolving around the ministrations of food by woman's hand? Could it also be that favorite food and the attraction to women correspond to the birth trauma of original denial? Could something sneaky and unsuspected be going on undetected because we regard the relationship as natural?

Fact: most people would find it virtually impossible to eat a steady diet of natural raw, uncorrupted food. Our fallen identities are not fitted for it. A piece of fruit as a treat, a token carrot, perhaps. But ask yourself, how long can you go without familiar steaming-hot conglomerations? Try living on cabbage, turnips, corn, fruit, and raw nuts for a while; see if your ego does not go into conniptions—feel as though it were being cheated of the regal portions of life it deserves.

Truly good food (and a truly decent woman) is an anathema to the male ego. Why? Because *only what is wrong excites and reinforces that which wrong excitement changed man to need.* Ego thrives on excitement and is attracted to the bosom nutrient of its recreation. Contact must be reestablished daily to the flow of ego life force from the parenting principle.

Here we are again; trauma changes us to need trauma as an identifiable earthy source. As I have said, the first thing the newborn gosling sees is its mother, and it will follow even a fox. So, there is the original establishing trauma, and then there is the romance with the fox. Then trauma goes on to reinforce and build what trauma established, and one day the farmer who has been kindly in fattening you through your needs is going to eat you like the Christmas turkey that you are.

Death stalks, awaits us all. We all come back to the kind of environment, the kind of food and women that traumatized and loved (hated) us as infants to be fattened for the kill. Your favorite food has little, if anything, to do with its being good for you. What I like, you may hate. It has to do with a conditioning need. A beautiful plate of spaghetti to an Italian has the same drawing power to pull him in as does an attractive Italian damsel, and both program him as an Italian. So the cultural person is not a person at all, but a mutation.

In order for the man of culture to evolve, his food and women must become more exotic and exciting—develop sophisticated, abnormal, kinkier forms of tease. Thus, soul progress lies in the adventure of the rebellious soul, wallowing in the glorifying lying spirit, penetrating ever deeper

50

through its acceptance into and beyond the forbidden zone. The journey through food and women (sex) is the rebellious soul's downward self-transcendence, and up comes an unholy self, standing in the place of the holy.

Rethink now. Do you honestly love mama's cooking because it is naturally, really, good; or is it because its nostalgic smells and aromas strengthen a sense of self, of worth, in you? Do you love that really *good* woman, or is a good woman, to you, one who allows you to wallow in lying affections, who reminds you that you are living, and not dying? Then let me remind you, woman was never designed for such support and other-self-indulgence. You will know something is wrong as you find yourself submerging deeper into women—you will even find yourself doing very strange things to crawl inside her or even food; you get into them, and something of them you *think* is you gets into you.

To tell the truth, you have probably never had a *natural* craving for anything! Compare the women/food thing with a drug addict's need. Food and sex are drugs—woman is the pusher and the fixer. Her ego appeal awakens the sex need, and then she fixes it.

Your favorite dish (or favorite tomato!) has little to do with what is *good*; rather, it has to do with what you have been *psychologically corrupted to need*—to crave. *Corruption awakens the need for itself in any form.* Remember when your mother wanted something from you, she made you your favorite meal?

Corruption, in drawing the soul down, awakens

the sleeping giant of sensuality; once awakened, your sensuality identifies the various awakened hungers as the way to go for fulfillment and escape from guilt. Sex is the first hunger awakened by the temptation of food. From then on, food and sex become an adventure to the soul's completion and salvation from having to face what has gone wrong.

But such consideration and false affections are from the very lying spirit that created us to need them in the first place. So you eat, drink, and have sex, and in so doing breed emptiness, dissatisfaction, and ever greater needs that can never really be satisfied. And the gratification of any need awakened by ego appeal is really escape and rejection of God to be God. The fall then breeds more need and, eventually, abject slavery.

Is there any doubt left that your destiny is being formed—with your will being controlled—through what you eat? Will you please at least consider this possibility? Then, are you the pusher or the pushover? What role have you been set up to play? *Men, you see, are conditioned to pressure women to be pushers and fixers. Women, feeling this pressure, respond—and that response spells their downfall into the animal life of man.*

Your identity was transmuted, and is presently sustained, through mama's presence and cultural food—with associated environmental objects and suggestions present at the time of corruption. In other words, an Indian is drawn to re-create his environment—his world. A skid row bum will take his world everywhere and establish it even in a

Madison Avenue penthouse. You can take the man out of the country, but you can not take the country out of the man.

Surely, cannibals are identifiable by what (or, rather, *whom!*) they eat. And cannibals elect cannibal kings, don't they? A king is dredged up—a lower being than those who elected him—to serve as a role model, to excuse and glorify the devolving cannibal selves.

Cannibal mothers have no tolerance for normal children; they are proud only of cannibal offspring, corrupting them with cruelty and rewarding conformity with love to make them become cannibals who grow up to need cannibal lovers and kings to reinforce the mama-propagated self in a familiar world of guile. So it is no accident that the woman you thought *you* chose to marry has the spirit of your mother, and her culinary arts are little more than sophisticated forms of corruption.

Anorexia has something to do with the recognition of food as being somehow connected to guilt—growing a guilt. Food first "saves" the ego as a friend in need and then is seen for what it is, a cause of guilt. The faulty logic is, if eating (to reject conscience) equals guilt, then, surely, not eating is the path to redemption.

Individual differences, conditioning, and suggestion make one person's mouth water for a plate of spaghetti, another's, for a cheese blintz. The common denominator of all our "loves" and cravings is association with individual and environmental trauma. We learn to "love" the person, the conditions, and the surroundings of our corruption.

As you "baptize" yourself in your romantic food and lovemaking with abandon, you are unconsciously reinforcing the behavior your mother set up in you through "her" presence in the experience.

Perhaps mother upset you as a child with her impatience, petty cruelties, and subtle, confusing power plays. You must have reacted with resentment, and the die was cast. Resentment awakened a sexuality and sensuality. Hunger, which is pejorative and regressive, which mother fixes and gratifies, is identified with more and more of "your" favorite food, more and more sex, and more gross acts by your wife or whore. And now whenever you are upset, you eat and have sex, and that is like getting closer to mother *and* her approval. The will of the woman and of the serpent is in every sex act and mouthful of food. And man's life is as a beast in a living hell. The tease of love or cruelty awakens the Beast to hunger for the teaser to fix. Do you see what this implies!

Women feel pressured by the men they can't help teasing, to keep them happy with sex, knockwurst, and pasta garbage, and men equate completeness and fulfillment and happiness with that. So, if you do what "mama" wills, then she gives you what she has made you want—food, sex. Men are donkeys. Manipulators scan rebels for established needs, serving them so as to rule. Thus it comes to pass that strangers take the place of honor of mothers and wives.

The goodies you crave are rarely simple and natural things, like a nice fresh apple or a carrot you could get for yourself and so not depend on the chef. An apple glorifies God. Apple strudel glorifies the woman. Through the strudel you are awakened to need, comes the will of the woman "god." Through the apple comes God (to the repentant soul).

Accordingly, it is best, if one is as wise as a serpent, and not so harmless as a dove, to invent a concoction, some exciting recipe hard to get or imitate that only mother or the dope dealer (or musician) knows how to make—hook us with it, so as to put a lot of willful self into it. A homemade cake, perhaps—something that would make you physically dependent upon that special touch—and then whenever she wants her way, she bakes that cake and withholds the cake or the sex till you are ready to meet her will. And you won't see what she is up to. Some women can do something special with cake the way no other women can do (and no other women will do!). A man corrupted by a whore's love will even give away his whole fortune to her.

The original "apple" has long since evolved into something infinitely more sophisticated—apple strudel! And innocent Eve has degenerated to become more glamorous females and whores, enticing and kinky. No matter what you give or what you do for them, they are never happy. They demand more and more, and you can't say no, can you?

It is an immutable fact that, once corrupted, a victim identifies emotionally, psychologically, and spiritually with the corrupter's ground of being and cannot exist apart from it. You cannot oppose "god," let alone *correct* her!

Set adrift from God, the image of God has faded for man, and woman's form obsesses his mind, instead. Alone on a desert island a shipwrecked sailor thinks and fantasizes about woman and food. He dreams away God and dreams about the god of his trauma-created being. The older and more corrupt a man is, the more his guilty mind focuses in a kinky way on woman to focus away from the awful truth of what he has become through her.

Pasta, as served by an Italian mama, reinforces the Italian male image; the Jewish identity is likewise fortified by a Jewish mama's matzo ball soup. (Believe me, you don't have to be Jewish to be a "Jewish" mother!)

I certainly don't wish to leave the rigid impression that you can never eat apple strudel or pasta again. You can—though it is not wise to do it too often—as long as you are careful not to abandon yourself in images and pleasure. Don't get "high" on it, in other words.

Failing that, every bite becomes a more exciting hypnotic fix, reinforcing the projected ego (mother) self of childhood which destroys the real man as it builds the false man.

Beyond the false image each foolish male has of himself, the image of the woman is secretly evolving in him. He is becoming effeminate, in other words. Through and beyond that, no matter how he may try to compensate through muscle and macho, male identity gives way to the devil himself; homosexuality and all manner of dark forces of perversion invade, and murder ascends from the pit of her embrace.

In other words, man is evolving downward; from man he becomes "male," from male he becomes a beast man—the devil's pawn—and finally he is completely pathologically possessed of the spirit of the serpent in the Garden. Evil's a psychopath!

What we see as "civilization" is really the rise of culture through the Fall of man. Culture and the ravenous, condescending love gods of culture appear to dominate man by displacing the soul that cries to God with a soul that cries out to hell in them. Culture is not civilization. It is a miniature hell on earth. Man exists on this earth hell as a beast-man lower order of being, with different loyalties and sustaining affections in a military chain of command, dominated by inferior beings in submission to Satan's spirits, commanders ruling through love and fear.

Let's touch again on how sex dissipation and enslavement are connected to food. The original trauma was oral—sin came by the mouth—first by the word and then by the food. Food causes the separation from God with the metamorphosing of divine being into animal being. Man is fixated to a woman's mouth, her form, her food. He ingests her spirit completely.

Man is compelled to return again and again to the scene of the crime. He craves to be corrupted, because corruption, to the sinner, is life-renewing and is self-creating. Through the love trauma, the selfish self appears; the imperfect ego self, gratified, is then perfected. Through such "love," the truth is denied, and the lie self is reaffirmed and takes form as the only reality and only true being.

Poisoned (altered) food is not only physical nourishment for the cultured (albeit inferior) self, but it also transmits deadly nectar to the spirit, a psychic stuff of which evolving infernal egos are made. For this reason even natural things and acts must be adulterated; otherwise, they cannot convey the vampire's spirit of eternal life from low-life love. Men's psyches have been altered to need this infernal life-in-death soul food—and the female's ego has been enlisted into the agony and ecstasy of providing it.

So, the food offering awakens man's sensual nature to lust, to collect worldly loves and experiences. The sin of forbidden fruit changed man to see woman not as a person to love, but as an object of extreme excitation and gratification. The worst in her called up to serve the worst in him. Food is responsible for change one, from nonsexual man to anxiety-ridden, sexual animal; the first female to "respect" and soothe the psychic embarrassment of the animal creates change two, addiction to false love through sex; thus, 1) false love through food, 2) false love through sex, and so on.

Each sin of gratification awakens lower, baser hungers to fix. The next sin of the need for acceptance (pride) appears (actually descends) as a symptom—a hunger—to be soothed, treated, and fixed. Sex is the symptom of failing, and when its embarrassment is fixed, that fixing, being a rejection of God, becomes another failing to embarrass and to be fixed.

Now we have 1) eating to forget the guilt of eating and 2) having sex to forget the guilt of having sex— leading to drink, and so forth. Every act is a denial of God and the destruction of the true man, awakening a base man as though it were a man-god in the process of creating himself.

Unconsciously men cohabit with their mothers. However, this point is not to be confused with Freud's well-known theory of the oedipal complex. It is more metaphysical in that men identify with the *spirit* of their mothers; their mothers' dominating spirit creates them, while the submissive, "understanding" female saves them and so sustains the order coming through mother.

Men are continually sizing women up, seeking in every one they meet the spirit of the mother they knew as a child. Little does man suspect that that is exactly how his father was destroyed and corrupted by his dominating wife and how his father became subject—and it's how, through the failing of every father, Original Sin comes down through the never ending chain of abused mothers.

Thus, every woman man marries is his mother (or grandmother); and his conditioning to woman's body is connected to the security of a female childhood violation of him, by way of his father's failing with his mother. Women even violate their male children at their breasts—getting some kind of sexual excitement from feeding and overreacting to their male infants and driving them into dependence.

A wife, then, simply completes what mother originated—kills him and goes on to dominate and corrupt the next generation of vipers.

Lousy cooking and a strong hatred for a dominating mother can compel men to select a wife who is not only a dominating hate object, but who is a terrible cook to boot! Why? Because the perverted sense of independence can be dependent upon having a woman against whom to rebel. The ego can evolve and flourish in a sense of freedom from hating a wicked woman just as much as from being loved by one.

So, he marries a nag in order to be "free" and evolve a will of his own, maintained by challenge, using her self-righteous nagging to do the opposite of right—as an excuse to justify being completely selfish and irresponsible!

For everyone there exists a hate/need relationship where love is simply use, where love's attraction has its basis in hate. "Love" breeds hate and hate, love, endlessly.

Beware! Rebellion against a wicked mother does not evolve you apart from her, but makes you the overt extension of her. What a damnable trick to become what you hate, to have the will you evolve become the will you opposed—and looking so wrong that the original evil seems to be saintly and saving and damning!

I have said before that hate is connected to "love" in the sense that through the guilt of resentment, the ego is sensually awakened to need the (evil) love of the hated object. As Adam blamed woman for his own failing, so was another love need born. Hate, blame, and judgment are as much a part of man's ego development as the stroking of "love" is. Both love and hate tease, puff the ego up and sustain it. Both love and hate evolve a self out of hell's corrupting power. Resentment and "love" are the two base legs of the ego triangle. Men fall to love and, through eventually seeing its betrayal, descend to hate and blame. Hell's hate then creates a need for hell's love endlessly.

Seeking love/hate fulfillment, man slowly evolves a devil, giving up real life to the seducer, becoming her dog of contempt; his only desire is to the false self as the true self, and he forgets reality by wallowing ever more deeply in the exciting muck of false love.

The spirit of the Fall, through woman, ascends to the family throne by pandering to male ego need, making of him the cripple and of herself the power, thriving on the miasma of her husband's decay.

Condescending female love dominance cripples and drives all men mad. Men have come down to need love, but when they get it, they feel violated, degraded by it. They feel *more* anxiety from relieving anxiety—like drinking to comfort the guilt of drinking, creating greater anxiety to drive one to drink. In a like manner does female ego security make for more insecurity.

The reason: exciting security is violent; "love" is violent and deceptive; it violates and degrades, making for greater insecurity as it is discovered.

Love is also perceived as betrayal, after the fact, so what satisfies and serves to evolve the dark side of our nature violates the other.

The immense excitement of female love penetrates and violates the sanctuary of man's soul and brings out the beast to pressure the woman. His lust and ego craving now penetrate her and violate the woman so she becomes a female. She is done in by the animal nature that her false love has brought out to love (lust) her. While woman corrupts and brings out the beast of lust, the Beast degrades the Beauty to serve it—a vicious cycle. Woman, then, became female through being violated by the lust her food offering brought out of the man. Her love must lie, and her lie changes him. His love (lust) violates her, causing her to become a supportive and lie-loving, whimpering dog of lust.

The female supporting principle always ends up by dominating; to serve the ego is to rule it. Male violence cannot restore a man's former authority, which was by grace. The woman's response to the man's violence is again submission to his ego, and all women who are forced to submit or who do so willingly, conquer the beast that tries to dominate them.

So, while man is mentally using and violating his woman sexually, she is outusing, outviolating him, making him over with lying love, shaping him into her image animal for her ultimate contempt. The Beast identity, now firmly established, draws completion for its ego by penetrating her mind, calling out hell—the perfection of his pride.

Women violate men with "love," men violate

women with violent sex; they mutually degrade one another.

The pride of most women denies that the love they are born to give lies, because lending support to man's betrayal of God is the source of woman's power. To assist man's rebellion against God is to become his god.

Understand, I am not blaming women for this state of suffering. They, too, are victims of failing fathers and violating mothers. Violating mothers set sons up to fail women, to give woman's god power, to know women as the spiritual completing of their fallen existence. And as they do, she is again violated by sex love and he is beguiled by her embrace. Yet, a woman can hardly have a relationship with any man without being a bitch and a liar, and the lying, manipulating bitch is the exciting trauma source that men recognize as a "proper" lover—for man's ego existence is based on the violation. An exciting lie made the rebellious ego exist subject to the betrayer's trust.

Responding to the call of the wild, the woman's spirit cannot help rising in a way that violates her beloved, implanting the lower order in him, which calls to her in a need that violates her again and again. And man, being violated sexually as he was once violated through food, cannot help but go on responding in need, with sex as with food—penetrating and violating her, drawing up the hell in her to trap him in a squirrel cage of doom.

Only when a man sees that he is outviolated by that which he violates, outused and outdominated by what he uses and dominates, can he begin to give up all his poisons, his lust-as-love, through which former pleasures his own substance was being eaten out by a life-draining, bloodsucking, female vampire spirit.

Unfortunately, most men see all this too late—most, never, ever.

So, what is the answer? It is this: All men must admit that their love has been perverted from its true course. And women must see that, too, and not be sorry for, or provide support to, men who are weak, wrong, and needful. For a man cannot love a woman he needs too much. Not giving such love *is* true love. Not hating weakness will keep a woman from the horror of loving that weakness.

Repent of the pride of ambition, of the illusions of grandeur that call up all the wrong helpmates.

The ambitious woman's acceptance of the wrong in man is the transforming sin of Adam and Eve. It is yours also. Woman's acceptance helps man rebel against God's will. It tricks him into accepting her will; and it turns out her will is not her will at all, but hell's plan for them both.

Still, because this writing has been so negative, I want to emphasize that I am *not* speaking in reference to natural affection and natural eating. Realize away the unnatural—and only the natural remains. Become objective with the harmful attitudes that pervert your relationship with food and love, and true love remains.

Observe away every wrong relationship, and your life will become a tempered balance, a natural and blessed experience.

CHAPTER 5

The
Jaded Palate

From the beginning, mankind has hungered to fill the void created by Original Sin, first with food and later with sex and other attractions. The trauma of Original Sin has created in us a void that cries to be fulfilled by the very thing that created it. We hunger and thirst, but nothing satisfies. The more we eat, the emptier we become. Something eats away at our substance with every mouthful. So it is not so much what we eat as what is eating us *as we eat* that needs examining.

The emptiness we all feel comes from our having fallen away from the true ground of our being to live another kind of life, a life that is contrary to the original design of our Creator.

The drug addict's fixation is similar to the one we all share with food. Drugs, like food, create a need for themselves, a hunger that promises fulfillment only if we continue to take them; but as you see, they deceive us, giving us illusion in exchange for our souls.

The corrupting power of Original Sin, its power

to suck out the victim's life essence, hinges on the principle of deception, the art of stealing life through trauma and emotional excitement—this, in the guise of *loving* or giving emotional support. Every fisherman knows that the only fish he can catch with bait is a very hungry one! So it is with man. In order to be caught (deceived) and reeled in, the "fish" must be hungry for, or compatible with, deception. We are excited and caught primarily by our own selfish, egocentric lusts and needs evolving from, and supportive of, the ego's rebellion against the spirit.

Now, the interesting thing about needs, as far as man is concerned, is that once he has been *caught*, an inordinate hunger for the bait begins to grow up in him. Each time he is hooked by the reaction of trauma, his emotional need for the bait is intensified; but unlike the fish, man goes out *looking* for the fisherman in order to get hooked. He seeks the excitement of tease as though his life depended on it—and in a sense, it does.

A man will surrender his real life to the corruptive process he calls *love*—to a hell disguised as heaven. He enjoys the struggle against being reeled in, and his resistance (resentment) makes him hungrier for the bait of love. Indeed, that hate actually makes the bait more attractive. Egotistical men love to hate, because hate literally creates the appetite for, and is compatible with, the spirit of beguilement. For the beast men, it is the only love and fulfillment they want to know. Gross, egotistical men equate their bigger appetites with evolving manliness.

You, on the other hand, may not ideally be a gross animal, wallowing in lust for ego fulfillment. Yet, your resentment of the game, the struggle, the challenge, that you see other men enjoying, will not help to free you from being caught fast by the love game yourself. On the contrary, your efforts to steer a safer course will only intensify your need to swallow the bait—hook, line, and sinker. Your preoccupation with the forbidden ecstasy will cause it to become increasingly attractive to you and more troublesome. Forbear, then, to let your weakness challenge you to do battle with it. If you do, you will find yourself creating, and then giving in to, the appetite you hate, and it will swallow you up.

In this game of life that degrades one into playing the role of predator or victim, what more subtle bait can there be than food? Food, like woman, can be both natural and seductive. *It is usually not until we have had a great fall and have become extremely troubled in the soul that we are ready to appreciate the fact that there is a difference* and that we stand ready to try to define it. But define it, we surely must, if we are to experience a right and natural desire for the truth that will make us free.

The trouble is that all the experiencing we revel in before we hit bottom and realize something is wrong produces in us a preference for the unnatural. Most of us have become so involved with worldly pleasure that the unnatural satisfactions have come to look like natural fulfillment to us. They are certainly more exciting, pleasurable, and satisfying to our egos than truly natural experiences, which have come to appear *unnatural*, uninteresting, boring, and even threatening to our egos.

The result? We focus our attention on the *salvation* of our unnatural lusts, seeking to make them ever more satisfying to our jaded palates that grow hungrier for that misidentified *something missing*, in spite of all our misguided efforts toward fulfillment.

Our tap water might be the purest in the world—no matter. Our sophisticated palates begin to demand *Perrier*. We may have been eating margarine for years, but when we hear Vincent Price say that *he* can tell the difference between margarine and butter, well, who wants to admit that his senses are less refined than Mr. Price's? We ascribe human attributes to wine, like "innocent," "unassuming," or "hearty." And so we carry on refining our tastes to the nth degree, and what does it get us? A greater emptiness, a greater longing for real satisfaction. The kind of fulfillment we have been chasing breeds only frustration, which is another form of challenge and resentment.

And resentment is the hunger connection—the sin that awakens the hunger we *love* to indulge.

Once we have become locked in to this senseless vicious cycle of fulfillment through the senses, however, it becomes very difficult for us to accept the fact that this kind of fulfillment is a thief, an enemy, and a betrayer. We think of pleasure as our only reward or happiness. Our emotional yearning grows so powerful that it bends our thinking into believing that any effort we might make to deny its appeal or even to struggle against it is a folly tantamount to going against our own true nature.

We are as easily manipulated by our own spiritual longings *as a fish is by its hunger* when we go about trying to satisfy them through things *out there*. And the fishermen of the world are always seeking new ways to make their bait more effective to gladden our selfish souls and keep us happy in our fool's paradise. Some fish develop enough smarts to avoid the bait, but not us! We entangle ourselves ever more deeply in our web of pleasure and despair, and from the depths of that despair, there rises a sensuous hunger, a burning fire demanding to be quenched with still more fire. It is a vicious cycle.

Soon after we are born, our natural spiritual hunger is altered and, in that impure state, amplified by longings that have evolved from some failing we have forgotten (and have no desire to remember). These longings evolve into unconscious yearning for all the wrong things. So we all unconsciously look at natural things in an unnatural way; witness the way men look at women, for example. Such looks can be frightening to an innocent girl, but once she has been violated by the lustful glance, she falls to become addicted to being lusted after.

What did Solomon say about the lusts of the eye, the ear, and the senses? He warned that they could never be satisfied by seeing, hearing, and feeling, for there is no fullness there.

You may agree with me in principle, but the hardest thing for me is to get you to perceive the unnatural way you look at everything. Now please look carefully at the events of your recent past. Rewind the tape of your memory, in a manner of speaking, to this morning or yesterday morning, and play it again.

Look at your reaction to the contents (or lack of same) of your mailbox, to the unexpected call you received (or expected but failed to receive), to the unexpected stroke of luck (or misfortune). Now don't you see how you react to everything you see, feel, hear, taste, and smell, with undue excitement? Your eye reaches out to fondle male or female forms and images. Your ear is ravished by the sounds of music (or what passes for it), by words of praise or of criticism.

If you observe a child at play, you will see how quickly his interest shifts from one thing to another, how short is his attention span. He is a perfect example of the true learning process in action. When he has finished his discovery in one area, his interest falls away and he goes on to the next adventure.

Wouldn't you be concerned if the child remained fixated, day after day, to his blocks or toy soldiers, fondling them, studying them, as though they were the be-all and end-all of his purpose on earth?

Yet men are fixated to women that way. They become so totally preoccupied with studying women, their image and form, that eventually a man's whole life revolves around discovering and growing through woman. But don't stop there—include music, drugs, alcohol, work—the list is endless.

So, to return to our basic subject matter, when your life begins to revolve around food, you must know that something is terribly wrong. You glorify your lust, your romance, your fixation. You write "love" songs about your sexual weakness. Through overreacting, whether openly or in secret, you sin. Your ego derives a great sense of pleasure and satisfaction as you wallow in your wakened senses. The *you* that is dying feels vibrant and alive again through the feelings that have been awakened by sin. Forevermore you must sin to experience the illusion that you are gloriously alive.

But in those moments of "unconscience," of "coming alive," death enters in, enlarges itself inside you, and leads you deeper into unnatural experiences for your sense of being alive.

It all began in the Garden of Eden with the fruit of the Tree of Knowledge of Good and Evil that was forbidden to us. This same fruit was the means by which evil could manifest *its* will. The forbidden could have been anything. It could have been a horse, for instance; ride it, and you are out of favor. It is disobedience that separates us from God's love, from the wellspring of the sensible life, and introduces us to the spirit of the sensual life, to a spirit of false love and reinforcement which enters through the quickened senses through doubt and through emotion. And what is sin but transgression of the law, of the will of God—the displacement of one will by another?

Sin is what psychologists refer to as trauma. Trauma is a response that shocks, seduces, and changes the foundation of our being, our very allegiance, what we believe and feel, the way we look at what is good and what is evil. Through it we begin to believe that evil is good! We begin to believe in our sin-awakened feelings, which, having been born of a lie, continue to deceive us.

So, Original Sin, or trauma, excited and changed man's allegiance; and his entire life began to revolve around the beguiling spirit of that change, manifested in an unhealthy fixation on food, women, and other forbidden delights. Thus, an unnatural longing for food and sex has been passed down through the mother by way of every father's failing since Paradise was lost.

For hundreds of generations, children have come into the world subject to the order of woman/food domination, an order devoid of true love and correction, an order rooted in the wrong kind of affection, the wrong way of reacting and taking false pleasure in the things of the world. *After the Fall the only love left in life for man was wine, women, and song, all of which he grew to enjoy in an unnatural way—the other love and way having been lost to him.* And all these things had to be made unnatural in order to give him a sense of fulfillment. Because such fulfillment also serves as an escape from what he is becoming through fulfillment, the sin serves two purposes: salvation from guilt and the evolution of the beast man as *god*.

So, women came to be admired for their beautiful wickedness, and food became bad (altered) in order to be *good* and desirable. Just tell your kids that a certain food is bad for them—forbid them to eat it—and immediately it becomes exciting and attractive to them, even if it is horseradish. Warn them not to become involved with this person or that, and you *know* whom they will turn to. You can see the danger, but all they see is *love* fulfillment.

Again I am asking you to reexamine your longings and yearnings. Ask yourself if the things you want really satisfy. If they do not—if they lead only to frustration and an intensification of desire—realize why you are hooked. Even as you indulge, you yourself are being eaten alive by the age-old food/mother/woman syndrome.

CHAPTER 6

Food:
The Beloved
Tyrant

How often have you eaten, knowing that it was bad for you? And how many times have you done something you knew wasn't right in your heart, but you ignored your conscience and went ahead and did it anyway? What does that tell you about yourself and your state of mind?

Surely, if you eat what you know is bad for you, food must represent some kind of rebellion. Eating that way is against your own best interest and what is truly good. But in your rebellious state, it will appear good; bad holds out a false promise of good.

What you may not realize is that eating for *freedom and rebellion* is also subtly connected to a selfish life of folly; even a life of crime can be related to the Twinkie fix. It is not the chemistry of food that does the trick as much as it is the wrong reinforcing what has gone wrong in us. Man eats the worst and is attracted to the worst to breed for the worst.

Man feeds and breeds the worst in himself, and that is how civilization declines. Of all the creatures, only man can do such a thing, and he is born under a curse and compulsion to do it to himself.

The original root of our word *diet* derives from the Greek *diaita*, which means "a manner of living," or lifestyle.

Theoretically, if the Fall of man was indeed by way of ego rebellion against the Father's will by means of eating a mind-expanding substance, a forbidden food, we would find the change of personality maintained by that same trauma to this very day. A compulsion with food and regressive degeneration would have transmitted to the entire human race. Look, and you can see that it has; look at others, and then look at yourself.

The *Bible* records that through one man sin *and* the entire human race came into existence. And it was through abstinence from forbidden food that our Creator made his will known. Be mindful, then, your willful rebellion is presently maintained by eating what is bad for you. A farmer will feed his prize bull the very best diet, but for himself, he will choose to eat junk.

Why should wrong food be more appealing, more exciting, more romantic, and more powerful an influence than your own conscience?

The answer is that the spirit of our fallen nature has control. The wrong spirit that has grown up in us through the trauma of rebellion has developed its own nature and needs and is evolving by indulgence. It recognizes the supportive spirit of the wrong in food as the answer to its need; and you think these desires are your own. They are not!

Any kind of trauma can reverse the polarity of

our souls and, consequently, our lives. Wrong that supports our personal selfishness has become the *life* for the rebellious self. The wrong things we eat give us a false sense of confidence in the wrong, selfish things we do.

We cannot eat what is good, simply because we won't. The right food sustains the right way, and the wrong food reinforces the wrong way as the right. Cultural food is a friend; it is the life of our rebellion. A prideful, willful, ambitious person cannot eat correctly, can't stop smoking or drinking or whatever, even though he knows it will kill him in the end. Giving up bad habits is a matter of attitude—basically, an attitude toward God. In the wrong state of mind, the only way to give up a bad habit is to trade it for another—like smoking to stop eating.

Any bad habit frees you to do what is selfish. It frees you from the inhibitions of conscience to reach gloriously, ambitiously, beyond your grasp. You can be a food, coffee, or cocaine achiever. The bad habit first traumatizes, then changes you spiritually, psychologically, physiologically at the core of your being. It adapts you to a life of selfish fulfillments and dependency to complete an evolving selfish pride. Pride, you see, *can evolve only by doing what is wrong* and sinful; if it isn't sinful, it is not exciting. Wrong is "good" for what ails you—for what has gone wrong.

So, the spirit of the traumatized "changeling" recognizes the spirit of sin that re-created it in its image in every experience beyond food; a spirit leads the way to glory, to perfecting our imperfect self through lower and lower experiences with perversity.

You eat to rebel, to be free to do whatever you selfishly want. And then you eat to deny any guilt; you eat to release yourself from the inhibitions of conscience and the condemnation of its guilt—to do wrong again to forget you did wrong. *You eat to forget.* And if you can't get a Twinkie fix, your ego will be in danger of remembering what a fool you have become. Food, like any other bad habit, is not only a *denial of God*, it is the embrace of evil as the ultimate good, and that is why it is like love. Your habit reinforces, justifies, *rewards* selfishness and wrongdoing. Its "love" excuses everything wrong with you so you feel falsely smug and *secure.*

Wrong food and strong drink represent the *life* and spirit of the willfully rebellious, and you cannot give up the embrace of the lifestyle that is killing you until you are ready to change your attitude.

Wrong food first corrupts a soul to crave wrong food to be rewarded with ever regressive, more exotically wrong concoctions. The more tempting food or anything else becomes, the more it represents an adventure of the soul.

That same ego-supportive food mother gave your dad she also gave to you as a child. She forced you to eat her poison. She became threatened if you turned your nose up at it, because that meant her will could not have its way through you. A willful mother cannot control a child who won't eat her concoctions.

The principle of never accepting candy from a stranger is the principle of never giving your will over to evil through a morsel of forbidden food.

The entire spectrum of tragedy revolves around being drawn like a moth to the infernal flame of an ego-supportive "mother" of fallen existence. What went wrong with man through woman cries out to be sustained by woman, first by way of food and later by sex.

And again the principle of sex through food is simply this: Trauma (eating wrong food) changes the nature of man from self-perpetuating being to procreating animal. All sin, through putting to sleep the awareness, awakens the sensual dark side of our nature and all the inordinate animal hungers. The eternal life principle of perpetuation by *regen*eration becomes perpetuation by *de*generation—sex is death made to live again; sin is a living death.

So forbidden food, acting as a supportive trauma agent, not only creates an inordinate need for itself, but violates as it comforts, thus causing another symptom—sex becomes lust and lust becomes perversion.

Every forbidden impulse produces its own symptom. Let us say, for example, you become upset and you get an ulcer. The ulcer, in this case, is the *symptom*, the devolutionary result of your responding wrongly. Overreacting with resentment *is* a sin of resentment and it even creates sexual impulses.

Some people have learned to remain sick to get sympathy. Here they get the ego love they have always craved and could not get in any other way except by being sick. So they learn to stay sick for love. And sickness, when "loved," becomes sexually exciting.

So are all men sick for love. Their symptom, the pain of it, is lust. The trauma of wrong food builds the ego self and eventually awakens stronger lust, which cries out for love. It is love that makes men lovesick animals—dying lovesick animals.

Fact: *Any trauma induced by either seductive violation or violent violation defers evolution to the animal nature and the dark side of the spirit. So that—no matter what it is that excites or upsets us—we awaken to the sexuality of lust and of gluttony. And when either of these is indulged, it becomes another trauma, the anxiety of which causes us to hunger with lust for food and sex. The frustration (resentment) of sex leads back to indulgence in food, and that leads right back to sex again, and the accumulating degeneration of all this love/hate trauma leads downward to the awakening of perverted and dark desires of homosexuality, child molestation, violence, and murder.*

Man's denial of God, his rejection of God, has created in him an equivalent need for the spirit of the female. As a child, man is violated by this female presence, and the wrong in him craves female reassurance through food. Spiced food is love and, moreover, is an adventure into the spirit of the female. But the main symptom of his fall through the woman is the awakened sensuality. At first blush, animal sexuality is an embarrassment to all men. Ignorant of its cause, they all seek sympathy for the "condition."

So, without realizing what danger lies ahead (except for a heart-racing fear to warn him at the threshold of first romance), he reaches blindly for love of a woman to cure insecurity—but that reaching acts as a denial of how embarrassment came into being. Now we begin the journey into hell. Not only do we have food problems, but we are evolving sex problems and other base desires. Every base desire as it appears, like homosexuality, breeds a reassuring need for relief and love and a need for a lowdown lie-lover.

The lower man sinks, the harder it is for him to face himself. He must get his perversion fix. We are attracted to people lower than ourselves for love, and ever more dark symptoms are awakened to need low-life lovers.

The ancient serpent (along with its modern counterparts) knew about the power of food to alter man and his destiny.

The lifestyle of a spider revolves around its habit of catching and eating flies. A cow's preoccupation is with grass, a koala bear's is with eucalyptus leaves. A cow would probably not be a true cow eating a steady diet of flies. Adapting would have it change its form, its habit, and its function. A fly-eating "cow" would not necessarily take a spider form, but neither would it be as it once was. To survive a severe change of diet, the form and function could well follow and that "addiction" to that lifestyle be indelibly impressed upon successive generations.

Perhaps I have made the point about man. I

conceded that man is omnivorous, surviving upon almost any food source; granted, man is not locked into grass or meat or insects.

With us, change (of lifestyle) is caused by a trauma, or sin. Sin has the power to downgrade our "evolution" and development. *Trauma* is the pseudonym for *sin*, and as you now know, trauma is what has impregnated pride in man and adapted him to need it.

Trauma altered man's identity at the core of his being and caused an evolution in his own lifetime. The root of that change, the cause of that trauma, is food. Food caused change, and it sustains change. Food and trauma are one and the same thing. Few people can eat food that is good for them. We are under a compulsion to eat the wrong kind of food, and as we do, we maintain our separation from God. We maintain our rebellion against reality, along with every strange psychotic quirk, failing, and bad habit. Our soul is addicted to the food that will mutate and kill us.

Through one man, sin and the entire human race came into existence; forbidden food is at the root of all, so that every bite reinforces the failing attitudes of ego and edges us closer toward a spiritual death *through a physical one.*

Look at the decadence, the fall of the human race. From youth trace a young man's downward self-transcendence into skid row. Look at photos of yourself as a young person and again when you are older and more decadent, and you will see a bizarre change—often you will see someone else looking back at you.

Every sin brings with it subtle and pejorative changes; the pleasure of every reinforcing trauma brings a little bit of unconscious sleep, and sleep is the brother of Death. Any exotic pleasure is the reinforcing trauma—especially food. Food is denial by compulsion, whereas it was once denial by choice. You are under a sentence of death, and you are merrily eating your way there.

The food trauma is the mind-altering drug of consciousness. Food helps us forget reality; and through our diminished capacity, we enter the realm of deception and, through deception, death. Through many denials, deceptions, and changes, we finally arrive at death. But then—the wages of sin was always death. *But we have never known the truth about sin.* We have never known the reason why we all inherit death as part of life. Food keeps us deceived so we cannot perceive the truth; the life of pride is really death. We perceive death and dying as life and living—food is the essence of this illusion.

Just so long as we are stubborn, that long will we be slaves to sin and death through what we put into our mouth. We will no more be able to give up our food fix than the drug addict can his drug fix.

Entire cultures are fashioned and sustained by their foods. Food was man's downfall, and food supports everything wrong with man and his culture. Cultures rise as the civilized man falls, with tyrants displacing God as the godhead of our conscience.

If I instructed my son not to ride his bicycle for his own good and a friend talks him out of that, he then falls from my grace. He becomes subject to his friend's enticement—comes under his power.

In much the same way, our creator Father made his will known by means of a tree and its fruit. Disobedience through food separated His son from the power of God, and that man's soul was delivered to the alien power, to a different "chief." The chief is our "beloved" tyrant. Now you understand the power of sin; it is trauma, and trauma is change—a change only God can save us from, through repentance.

Food sustains the trauma "life" of sin, man's rebellion against God (good), and delivers him to the guileful spirit of a female. Woman stands behind the food, and the spirit, behind her form of rebellion. The willful person goes back to mama for consolation just as a naughty kid gets ego support from doing mischievous things with all the wrong company. But then he is rendered dependent on his friends for the animal delusion of freedom, for the feeling of righteousness, and for the direction of his ambition and his pride.

The spirit of food violates and, after it has violated, becomes a lover, a friend in need, a necessary evil for the lies our soul is dependent on. *The lie is the root of our fallen being*—our stubborn pride needs the escape, the consolation, to survive.

Yet, the fix leads to more fear than it cures; to fix an anxiety, it becomes necessary to sin, to indulge, to escape into food!

All violating objects of power have this one thing in common: that after their wickedness shocks and alters the form, they then become the necessary evil, loving, seducing, *serving* the altered form until the day of its death.

Thus, there is only one basic trauma, only one point where one is normal one moment and mutated the next. And once impregnated with that change, the changeling then cries out for the mother of its existence to nurture it with a sick love. And *food* is mother's love.

The love of food is the love of corruption, a wolf in sheep's clothing. Wherever there is forbidden (cultural) food, there also lingers a female presence. Food is a reinforcing, supportive symbol, like a flag.

Remember the rule that whatever is abhorrent and frightening before a trauma can become attractive and necessary for the new life after the trauma. Through food, then, we reinforce the spirit of the deceived self that got inside us; the love of food represents the devotion of a self-serving evil spirit. The lust for food and women represents an ongoing pride of man in rebellion against God.

In the same way that an alcoholic uses drink in an obvious fashion, so does a "foodaholic" use food less obviously to deny reason and shame.

We use food and sex to make contact with the spirit of our rebellion against God. And the sin of food goes on reducing our consciousness, gradually, imperceptibly, changing our character and lifestyle downward.

The female influence in the absence of the male

in the animal kingdom does not present a problem to the young, because no temptation or trauma influence exists for them. Only spiritual trauma effects instant change. Animals do not adapt or evolve in their own lifetime. Conditions select survivors, and survivors breed their differences.

Only man can evolve (devolve) in his own lifetime, and devolution came through a spiritual choice, to love God and to unfold as a bright-natured child of the light—or to reject Him; the trauma of the forbidden fruit altered mankind and caused a lie, death-centered existence, to become his lifestyle.

One man sinned, and through that man, the entire human race came into existence. *And the payment of sin is death.*

In the animal kingdom, then, there is no mind/ soul-altering female influence, and because there is none, there is no need for male counterinfluence. But with the man child, there is a need for a countering father influence, without which the female mutational influences of Original Sin project and carry forward into successive generations.

The male principle is from within, above; the female principle is environmental and from the spirit below. Man and woman represent two different kingdoms, two worlds, two dimensions, two systems: good and evil—two different lifestyles and evolutions.

Unfortunately, man is born inherently subject to the female principle. So he must seek the truth to save him from the woman's order of love before he can save the woman from herself.

A woman cries out for true love to save her from herself, and only a man who understands this real need and loves her (forbears to use her to build his ego) can save her. Only a man who has found God's love, who is *in*dependent and inwardly fulfilled, who has no need for woman's approval, can save— love—his wife.

But the whole man, the man who has found his way to real life, signals strength and independence and earns the respect of the woman. And it is the presence of God in man—the presence of goodness and justice—that awakens respect, and love joins her to the man who is reconciled to God. One cannot have respect for what is not respectable. Respect, love, and faith, then, are awakened by the actual presence of what is respectable. Love is born in the woman from beholding and experiencing the love object.

The *true* love of man for woman is the catalyst to the love from a woman, and her response *joins* her to him and separates her from a living hell. But male use joins man to the woman, reverses life, and her spirit then begins to govern and move up through generations.

So everything that has gone wrong with the human race hinges on a matriarchal existence, the surrender of man, the joining of male ego to a woman's reassuring love.

If life is not to be a living hell, the center of love in every home must descend down through the man, and not up through the woman. A woman can truly love only a man who forbears to use her.

The less a man needs a woman, the more independent he is of her; the more complete he is within himself, the more a woman is apt to respond with such love as few women have ever experienced. Women know (when they are needed) they are being used; they feel men calling up ugly hell out of their soul. And the hatred of man—the cultivation, the exploitation of his weakness—is recreated again and again until death do them part.

CHAPTER 7

The
Hidden Hunger

Have you ever found yourself standing in front of an open refrigerator, vaguely searching for something to satisfy an even vaguer craving, half knowing that you are not likely to find it? What if I told you that what you are seeking is a redeeming "presence?"

The presence you seek in the refrigerator is whatever it is that got into you by corrupting you, displacing your original presence of mind and standing as your god in its place. Both the original presence of mind and the substitute represent an intelligence, a life force, a stimulus to move and to be, except that one of them lies and debilitates, substituting illusion for the real meaning of existence. What you are seeking, standing there in front of the refrigerator, is something that got into you through an association with food—something that you identify as a remedy for anxiety, boredom, guilt, the sense of dying. You identify food with this intangible "loving" presence, and the effect is reassuring. Almost as good as the real thing. But not quite.

Presence of mind is the original life support, or "turn on" for man. Today, that presence haunts us as conscience, the conscience that too many of us regard as a useless appendage, something left over from a prehistoric era, something to be disregarded, or better yet, discarded. So what you are really seeking as you stand there is a kind of redemption through unconsciousness, or forgetfulness of conscience.

The compulsion that keeps drawing you back to the refrigerator is one you inherited from your mother's presence by way of the failing of your father. You are not likely to have escaped this compulsion, for all fathers have failed all mothers since the first mother offered the means of rebellion to her man. Men have eagerly sought this mothering presence from the beginning of time, so much so that this is the kind of love we regard as the norm.

Adam fell for the temptation because it offered him a chance to get out from under God's command and take on the godhead himself. But he swallowed the lie along with the food, and to this day, all egos depend on food for the sham "reality" it provides. We literally *eat* evil.

Suppose you have a son who gets caught up with a wrong crowd, goes out one night, and partakes of a mind-expanding drug. From that point on, you will no longer recognize him. His entire personality will be altered; his allegiance, also. He will no longer be your son. He will reject your love and have no interest in your forgiveness. He cannot, or will not, be sorry. He will have become your enemy, while the real enemy has become his "friend." And of course, his new "friend" will always be there to supply him with the substance of his corruption. As drugs corrupt, they also alter the identity of their victim to need the reassuring presence of the spirit of corruption.

The drug addict simply identifies the source of his (re)creation as the source of his reassurance. In his case, it is a drug. In the case of most of the rest of us, it is food, the original drug. As you lose yourself in its aroma, its color, its texture, you reinforce your belief in its false promise. You must surely see that if you allow yourself to be corrupted by anything—say, junk food, if you are a rebellious kid—it acts on you as a drug. You use it again and again, first, to reinforce your "right" to do it, and then to deny that there is anything wrong in what you are doing.

Food, unless it is grossly and morbidly misused, is certainly not the worst of all the addictive, destructive substances, but it is surely the most subtle. Both historically and personally, it is the first thing we fell to, and it forms the foundation for all the sins that followed. Because the need for food is so basic, and of such long standing, the many ways in which we have been misusing it are difficult to detect, and most difficult to cure. It will probably be the last problem we will ever solve, but it certainly is not the least.

The first food sin gave birth to lust, and then to hate. Like anything else that strokes us in some way, first, it pleases; then, we simply *must* have it;

finally, *damn* anything that comes between it and us. (Or fails to fix it just the way we want it—the way mother fixed it, of course.) Whether it's food or weed, we aren't addicted to it until we experience it, but once we experience it, something of the experience itself gets into us and cries out for the constant repetition and renewal of its essence. The drug addict doesn't cry out for chocolates, simply because his fall to addiction was not by way of chocolates.

Evil enters our souls through a forbidden substance, makes itself at home in us, and awakens our sensuality; so it is not only the forbidden substance (junk food, cultural food, liquor), which destroys our body, that we have to reckon with, but something evil that enters through the experience and eats away at our souls.

Case in point: You drink to deny guilt. But the drinking produces more guilt to deny. So you drink more heavily to deny the greater guilt. We follow the same pattern with food. The spiritual connection is quite obvious in many eating disorders, where we see the victim growing guiltier with every mouthful he takes to escape his guilt. Obviously, he isn't just upset over his gaining weight. Something else has gone wrong, something pertaining to the soul. So he eats and gets hungrier; he drinks and gets thirstier. Guilt has awakened his appetite for the substance of denial; and if he indulges his guilty craving all the way, it can lead only to his physical and spiritual death.

And how do you feel when you finally become

aware that the thing you love (lust after) has hooked and betrayed you? Your "love" turns to hate, of course. But hatred merely intensifies our lust. All alcoholics, food-aholics, and nicotine-aholics have a love/hate relationship with the thing they are addicted to, and it aggravates their need for the "love/hate" object.

I have often said "you can rebel against God, but not against the devil." We just enjoy hating too much to want to give it up. For one thing, hating increases our sensual appetites. When you hate something, the guilt of hating intensifies your need for the reassurance of the hated object. The love/hate relationship underlies all our human dilemmas. It even affects our striving, or refusing to strive, for material success. When we strive to succeed, we are often doing so in rebellion against a feeling of emptiness or inferiority that was laid on us in childhood by our "loving" parents or teachers. But with this motivation, any satisfaction breeds dissatisfaction, and we feel compelled to work harder and harder for fulfillment, until we keel over from exhaustion, with fulfillment still out of reach.

Hate expresses itself in the emotions of dissatisfaction, disillusionment, frustration, and often, merely in a futile attempt to find the emotional strength to rebel and overcome. But there is nothing we can overcome with hatred, because once we have fallen to it by way of the forbidden substance, we enter the realm of evolution. That is to say, whether we respond to evil with "love" (lust) or hate, we evolve in its image. You become what you love, and you become what you hate.

A normal person can have a glass of wine with his dinner, or in some social situation, without giving it a second thought, but the alcoholic can not. One drink leads to another, and another, until he has drunk himself into oblivion. He can not drink without denying and escaping reality. Likewise, the person with a food problem can not dine without denying. The problem is not genetic; it is spiritual. The lust for anything at all is a journey away from reality via the sin-awakened appetite.

Any overreaction to stress (temptation), whether it be a seductive or a destructive stress, separates us from the ground of our inner being. It wrests the true self from its reliance on the ruling love within, and replaces it with an alien identity that cries outwardly for the violating presence of the ruling spirit that spawned it. If the sin entered through food, the alien identity will be drawn to food like a baby to the mother that gave it birth.

The reason we are all so compulsive in our sinning is that the freedom to choose between good and evil has already been used up. The choice has already been made. When Adam chose to be his own god, the trauma violated him and tore him and his progeny from God's ground, once and for all. From that point on, all our "choices" have had to be compulsive in order to sustain our fallen, rebellious condition. We have to eat what is killing us, like it or not. All choices have to involve a lustful journey away from reality toward the fulfillment of our selfish pride.

The smoker may claim that he smokes because he wants to, and he may even think that he is telling the truth. But he is simply looking on his compulsion to ruin his health as his "free-will" choice. That way, his ego never has to admit that it is a slave to sin and death.

If you are able to resolve the hatred that amplifies your lust for anything, and which has grown from the original food sin, you will notice a very peculiar thing about your eating habits. You may already have noticed that the more you lose yourself in the aroma and flavor of the food, the more you will eat, and the more you will want to eat. Conversely, the less you eat, the less you need to eat. What enables you to eat less, of course, is the fact that you are hanging on to your consciousness and not allowing yourself to get carried away by your mouth-watering delight in the food. The more you are able to overcome resentment and return to the original presence of mind, the better able you will be to modify your reactions to the ego appeal of food in a spiritual way. As you grow in grace, you will see an improvement on both fronts; the thoughtful overcoming of resentment will result in a diminished craving for food, and the decreased consumption of food will gradually return the appetite to the normal service of the body that God must have intended. If, indeed, he meant us to eat at all!

Possibly, and this is only a conjecture on my part, we should be able to exist without eating at all. Christ once remarked, "I have food to eat ye know nothing about." His food, he said, was to do the will of his Father, not his own. Although he asked that we all become perfect, even as he was perfect, he obviously didn't expect his injunction to go over with the masses like a Springsteen album, inasmuch as he provided the multitude with loaves and fishes. And for all we know, the perfection we are meant to attain to would not involve a complete overcoming of the need to eat.

But even in the short run, experimenting with food and the conscious eating of it will prove that just remaining conscious at all times will not only give you control over your food choices, but will help you to overcome all your compulsions. You will gradually be redeemed from sin, able to make right choices endlessly. But even in this relative victory, you will soon discover that your choices are not of the original, pristine variety, inasmuch as Adam made the original choice for us. So the choice that is left to us is itself a kind of compulsion, but at least it is a salvation from the inheritance of wrong choosing. Our choices at this stage constitute a kind of reverse denial, a turning back from lust toward the redeeming light.

Why did Christ instruct his disciples at the Last Supper to eat the bread and drink the wine while remembering him? As I have often said, it was to reverse the effects of the original sin through which man ate while forgetting God's commandment. In other words, he was exhorting those who loved him to hang onto their consciousness and not lose themselves in tasty delights. Just see how the entire human race is eating, drinking, and sexing itself into oblivion. We just disappear, completely lose sight of ourselves, in the appetite that claims us; we lose our identity as we munch merrily away.

The moment you discover the gateway to the original presence, and choose to go that way, you become, in the words of Paul, "temperate in all your ways." All your appetites are gradually and effortlessly modified. All the things your ego lusted after begin to lose their appeal, and you begin to relate to people, places, and things with a new kind of mastery. Where before, you sought to possess, and ended up *being* possessed, now you will no longer seek to possess; yet, in a mysterious way, you will come into possession of the greatest gift of all, namely, control of your own life.

See how the food sin pulls you away from the inward sustenance of God's love and renders you void. And see how that in turn sets up in you a need to compensate with the nearest physical equivalent. Food is fulfilling in its way, and it feels like love from an original source. But your unholy delight in it sprang from an outside temptation, and it is the unholy spirit attending it that awakens and sustains your sensuality.

Alcoholics, in the last stages of their illness, look on their bottle as their one and only faithful friend and redeemer. What they see is a comforting presence within and beyond the bottle they hold in their hand.

When we live, as most of us do, in a decadent environment, we find it difficult to break free from our self-destructive habits because the mere presence of all those spirit-invaded people, places, and things almost compels us to partake of them. Our very conditioning, our codes of conduct, and rules of etiquette tend to hand us over to them on a silver platter. Their offerings have fashioned your soul by reason of your choiceless need to complete the spirit of pride they planted in you. You cannot reject whatever it is they offer to sustain your ego and keep it hooked to the forbidden substance.

Indeed, if you were suddenly to be cut off completely from your earthly delights, you would react like a bull in a china shop. You would go out of your mind with frustration and thrash about aimlessly, trying to collect your kingly "due" from everyone you bumped into.

Men are especially prone to violence where their sexual fixes are concerned. Their own resentment of the woman who denies them sex resentfully intensifies their craving to the point of desperation and violence. Denial of the "fix" threatens the ego with the horrible prospect of having to wake up to the truth of its enslavement.

The love men are addicted to has nothing to do with choice, but is a compulsive need for the lying love of sensuality. It is a towering, sustaining passion. Like true love, it reigns over man with absolute authority. The big difference is that true love is not sensual at all. The person who has found true love knows better than to seek it from anything in the outside world. It is absolutely non-needful and non-using of people and things. And it is despised by the world. How people will hate you if you dare to represent that divine presence they are running from!

Just as the drug addict needs and craves the presence of the mean-spirited drug dealer, so does an ordinary man need the presence of the food server. Men marry the women in whom they can identify the presence that was in their mother, the spoiling, serving, enabling spirit, creator and nurturer of pride.

The presence of a mean-spirited, falsely-loving female is very reassuring to a fallen, also mean-spirited male. He must fondle and stay constantly in touch with her form, even with her nagging spirit, in order to forget he is a dog, the reverse of what he likes to think he is, and be reminded that he really *is* some kind of god, as he worms his way into her and into the spirit beyond her.

The presence of the reassuring spirit in a person, place, or thing (a fresh apple won't qualify here, but a tasty strudel will, for sure) is compulsively accepted by the victim. Do you see now how a woman of easy virtue can have just about any man she wants and completely control him, while a good woman holds out no such promise to his advantage-taking ego?

Remember, once the choice to sin has been made, the power to resist sin is gone forever. The more we indulge, the more our foul spirit is "saved, completed, fulfilled!" The sinner is an opportunist; he will sell his mother for a fix. He looks for salvation in all the wrong places.

True salvation involves reconciliation with the

original Presence, the God from whom we became alienated through our disobedience. The fallen man has completely lost touch with true salvation. He looks instead to that other redeemer, the one that will "save" him from the Light and the awareness of his folly.

Remember, the very presence of any offering causes us to take refuge in it and draw on it compulsively for ego fulfillment. If we happen to become aware of our compulsiveness, we may try to rebel against its power over us by hating it, but hating it only makes it more attractive, if not in its original form, in another. That is, if you flee the presence in the woman you have come to hate for her mastery over you, you will soon be captivated and captured by the same spirit in another woman. If you take up smoking as an escape from your addiction to food, you will soon become just as compulsive to the spirit of nicotine. They constitute one and the same presence. That is why your answers to one problem soon evolve into becoming your next problem, and each substitution involves you more deeply in the process that leads to death.

The mere proximity of a woman can cause a man to fall in love—choice has nothing to do with it. It is compulsion. Her presence, like the golden, juicy turkey on the Thanksgiving table, awakens his appetite; and when she indulges him, her dark side not only welcomes him, but gets more deeply *into* the fabric of his being with every "bite."

When a woman signals acceptance by her looks, her manner, her very presence, the male ego falls to her subtle blandishments and his bodily senses are aroused. Her acceptance causes him to fall, which is another way of saying that it separates him from the inner ground of his being and awakens sexual hungers. As he gratifies his sexual hungers, he is compensating pridefully for what he has lost inwardly.

Food indulgences lead eventually to sex, sex indulgences to rage, rage to emptiness, emptiness to insecurity, and insecurity to greed for money. And it all starts at mother's breast.

Sex domination of a husband leads to female domination of the home, so that while food is not the immediate villain, the emotion it inspired *is*; and because emotion separates a man from his ground of being, it awakens hungers and lusts. When a woman dominates her male child and the boy reacts by resenting his father for not protecting him from his mother's tease, and he also resents his mother's mean or seductive spirit, his reaction separates him from the God spirit that should overshadow his father and subjects him to the female god presence. Thus begins his odyssey of addictions, from the simple food hunger through sex, drugs, alcohol, and music. Have you ever noticed how mother, having upset her child, consoles him with food, and thus conjoins her will to his through food forevermore?

I am not saying that food, sex, or anything else, is necessarily a sin, but until we have rediscovered our original ground (presence of mind) and fulfillment, we can not help but draw out of substances a mean sustaining spirit of death and tragedy.

Try simply being aware of the food in your mouth as you eat, rather than allowing yourself to get caught up in a flavorful dream state. The dark spirit that attends the world of imagination, when it is present in certain types of women, beckons with the promise of instant party time, and man is helpless. His mind, his body, his hopes for the future—all are sucked into the abyss. What he experiences is not a natural appetite, but a morbid enslavement to the object of arousal. He betrays all that is good in his life for the evolution of his selfishness.

The presence of a man draws up in a woman the compulsion to serve him. And in the presence of a woman, the man falls toward what his need compulsively draws out of her to serve him. Men and women are locked into one another in a vicious cycle of creating and serving each other's hell. They are compelled to destroy each other through their love/hate offerings. Men fall in lust, and women fall in hate. To a man, the spirit presence of a woman and everything connected with her—her clothes, her lips, her food, her nagging words, her spoiling love—is charged with a nostalgic essence.

Everything connected with the sin of sex takes on something of its aura, so that even the bed can become a sex object. Articles of feminine apparel, especially undergarments associated with the seductive woman, become charged with the power to awaken sexuality. A sleeping male has erections all night long. That is because he unconsciously takes comfort in his bed and in sleep. As a matter of fact, any reduction in consciousness can result in sexual arousal. Remember this fact whenever you find yourself "turned on" for no apparent reason. At such a time, a few minutes of meditation can help you get back on center.

A shameless woman is an infectious, unconflicted being. Such a person has the power to release a man from his inhibitions and get his juices flowing. She has had that power from the beginning. She acquired it first by appealing to man's desire to be god, and she hung onto it by catering to his constantly-reappearing ego/sexual needs. After all, a woman without shame, without conflict, sheds an aura of innocence over the delights she offers; as a result, the man feels that simply by coming into her presence, he will also partake of her apparent innocence and shed his burden of guilt.

The same principle underlies the power of tyrants. First, release the victim from the inhibition of conscience, create sensual appetites; then, offer salvation through false love. When we merge sensually with a ruthless, shameless person, we feel that we are buying release from our own guilt. You see, don't you, how easily we are tempted to identify with a ruthless, shameless, sexually-uninhibited person. Such a person seems to throw a blanket of innocence over everything we do with them; but there's a catch to it. Once we start buying release from conscience in this way, the price keeps going up, and we fall victim to more illicit passions and ambitions.

Kindly note the common thread running through the *modus operandi* of recent cult leaders. Jim Jones,

Charles Manson, and the Rajneesh all used free un-inhibited sex to establish their control over the "flock." It was the cement that made them "one," closer than blood kin; and at the same time, the sin stimulated guilts that had to be assuaged with still more sin, greater lust for more sexual salvation.

All feelings of guilt and failure, from whatever source, draw to the mind fantasies of salvation. In the case of men, the fantasies involve sex with shameless, unconflicted lovers; alone on a desert island, a sailor dreams of his favorite foods and beautiful women. And when we find our dream girl, we are aflame with a self-perpetuating passion, a growing need for love and sex that can never be satisfied. Then one day, should we discover that our lover is our destroyer and enslaver, we become violent and beat her into the ground, verbally if not physically, pick her up, make love to her, beat her, and make love to her.

Women, on the other hand, when they are frustrated by their inability to control or be controlled by a man, tend to look for comfort in food. Often, the woman who is constantly stuffing herself is feeding her male identity, derived from having interacted resentfully with a fallen man. The male identity that has got inside her teases her to feed and console it. Sometimes it works the other way in a male; his feminine identity teases him with food, so that he becomes his own chef, his own mother, as he insists on preparing his own food.

In both cases, sexual fantasies are awakened and indulged. The transvestite gets into his mother's identity via intense imagery and excitement induced by masturbation. He takes on her identity completely in order to avoid realizing the truth about himself.

One day you may discover that you can overcome your sex-based personal tragedies simply by eating sensibly, for the right reasons, from the Lord's table. What seems so natural and innocent at first, a wrong relationship with food, soon leads to sexual problems, and from them, to the abuse of every imaginable substance. By getting more and more into the substance, we not only buy reassurance for our ego, but we escape the realization of what is existing in our mutating, dying being.

Losing ourselves in anything, like the flavor of food, is like becoming part of, being embraced by, something greater than ourselves. It is the way we evolve our spiritual identity. As the Christian hymn puts it: "Let me hide myself in thee." The soul cries out to be absorbed, protected, and validated by its Creator. Is it possible to express a greater love? A greater commitment? Unfortunately, since the fall, our egos have been crying out with the same intensity, but to lesser gods—and have been taken in by them too. We cry out to the sinister presence behind our addictions to redeem us and to convince us that we are perfect just the way we are. Our sensual loves seem to absolve us of our faults. They rescue us from the need to repent of our sins.

At this point, if you have come to see the folly of your addictive ways, it would be wise just to drop all your relationships and hobbies without bothering to hold them up to your new light for re-evaluation. Anything you like or hate too much is likely to be the means by which evil is coming into your life from below. Just remember that what you are *into* is into you. You cannot escape into anything for refuge without identifying with the spirit on the other side of matter.

The spirit of the pure intellectual is of pride, and not of original understanding. It is not surprising, then, that the fallen man is reborn through what, for want of a better name, is an intellectual spirit, and the first offering of food is to the ego by way of the intellect. We embrace knowledge so that we might become wise as God is wise. Now, we are into knowledge, and the spirit of knowledge is into us, guiding the human race to individual and collective disaster. Incidentally, intellectuals are the easiest persons to corrupt. Entire nations are most often undermined by their intellectuals. And what is keeping the spirit alive?

The cunning of the intellectual spirit operated originally through food; so the pride of man continues to be sustained through food and the presence of women who know how to use food as the way to a man's heart. Just think of the nostalgic effects you experience in the presence of food, women, wine, and song. Your perverted soul, guilty as it is, has a boundless appetite for mind/soul expansion.

The guilty soul is an opportunist. It seizes on every offering to complete its identity of pride. It takes its gratification whenever and wherever it can get it. It is not to be trusted. It is a soul evolved from forbidden delights.

Everything that was present in the moment of the original trauma goes into the soul's memory bank, so that even the smallest bit of pertinent data will evoke the original excitement as surely as the homing salmon will return to the place of its spawning. Thus are even the most disgusting habits of thought and deed constantly reinforced.

The food on your plate wafts out its message: "Eat me, escape into me, forget your troubles and find your fulfillment in me." Sex delivers the same message. So do drink, drugs, and music. And each time you give in to your tempters compulsively, you draw from them more of the guilt-plagued identity that will keep demanding the substance of escape for its fulfillment. Of course, you tend to see your slavery as a form of devotion, like a glorious love affair. You see everything in a strange light; your friends become your enemies; your enemies become your friends.

Remember this important truth. We are descended from original sin, and thus, we are *not* free moral agents. We live under a compulsion to complete the journey of pride all the way to the hell that looks like heaven to us until the pain of our "choices" causes us to seek the truth that would make us free. The journey began at mother's bosom with her "love," and though you might rebel against mother's love, you will surely seek out her spirit in another woman who will finish what mother started.

You may flee from one compulsion, only to seek

out the same dark spirit in another form. It's a vicious cycle, because whatever helps you to deny God *is* your god, and it lurks within every symbol of your rebellion, even in something as innocent looking as a candy bar. It is not sugar that causes and maintains aberrations of character in "hyper" children. Rather, it is the reassuring spirit of pride that kids need to support and justify the wrong emotions that are churning inside them.

We have been re-created by the essence of temptation through substance abuse, and when the simple excesses begin to pall, we seek out something more sophisticated to give new life and energy to our jaded appetites. The dark side is always at hand, baiting us to open the door and make it welcome. And when it gets inside us, it cries out in our name with a growing lust.

Pride has a spiritual appetite all its own. Our fall from God to be our own god, through knowledge, has separated us from the original ground of our being and has rendered us void, lonely, insecure, dead. We try to compensate for our growing hunger (there is no end to knowledge, you know; who can hope to know it all?) through our senses, and for the most part, we take pride in all our failings.

Stop here for a moment, and reflect on the way you compensate for inferiority feelings with knowledge, food, and sex. You can become a knowledge-aholic, because the more you get into the spirit of knowledge, the more the spirit of pride gets into you. Do you see how you use knowledge to deny that you are stupid and inferior? To deny the truth?

You may acquire vast stores of knowledge to help you with your denial of truth, but you will wind up with less understanding along with a greater guilt.

Food constitutes the original temptation, the door through which the spirit of ambition, of being good through knowledge, entered our consciousness. For that reason, you must not lose yourself in the taste, the ego-sustaining flavor of food. Of course, because the lust for food and the lust for knowledge are so closely connected, you may feel a little stupid and forgetful of facts that are important to your ego as you start to modify your intake of food and to desist from emotional excitement, but don't let strange feelings of emptiness weaken your resolve to hang on to your consciousness for dear life. Do *not* travel down the pleasure path to stimulate your intellect. Do *not* travel away from the present moment by way of intense study or any other indulgence of your ego's dreams of glory. In other words, do not use food, sex, or anything else to stimulate prideful hopes and visions. Do not be lulled intellectually into a false sense of security; for the "sense" of security that you can obtain through ego indulgence is utterly false. It leads only to a greater hunger for knowledge, a greater longing for the people, places, experiences, and things that can never satisfy, but lead only to frustration.

Haven't you noticed that the more you allow yourself to get carried away by pleasure, the emptier you feel at the end of the road? Stubborn Pride says, "Go for it—let nothing stand in your way!" But if you go that way, you will wind up with more emptiness, more insecurity, more hopelessness, more guilt. And if you are not careful, you will find yourself taking the same futile trip again and again in your effort to escape the letdown that never gets any better, but instead provides the impetus for the next miserable "escape."

Therefore, be warned. Perish forever all egotists who enter here. Travel back to Reality through the practice of moderation in every thing you do. "He that striveth for mastery is temperate in all his ways." Become aware that you exist, and that you are merrily munching yourself away from Reality to tragedy and death. Get back on the right road by practicing the presence in every thing you do.

Be aware of yourself as you eat. Stop dressing up your food with spices and spicing up your sex for increased feelings of ecstasy. Feed all your appetites with caution and discretion, remaining aware of your tendency to overindulge them as a means of escape.

Only your utmost awareness and objectivity can keep you from floating off on the cloud of flavors and sensations to the dark side of your nature, to evolve as something less than what you were meant to be. Moderation, through awareness, detoxifies the system, enabling you to see more clearly by the light of Truth. This is the light that will drive out the prideful spirit and give you dominion over your soul and destiny.

CHAPTER 8

The
Last Supper

A wild beast, having no ego to feed, rarely—if ever—overeats. Man, on the other hand, thanks to the sin of pride, has descended so deeply and guiltily into his animal nature that he now finds it virtually impossible to feed his physical hunger without at the same time satisfying and reinforcing the ego cravings of his descended being.

To become temperate in your ways, you must find the way to give up ego involvement with your food. Surely, the ultimate fast is not food denial, but ego denial, and you may well ask: How is such a thing possible? The weakness for food that has been imparted to us, encouraged and condoned by our culture, has become so much a part of our lifestyle that few of us come to know the joy to be found in triumphing over the ego's involvement with food as a source of pleasure. Test it.

See if you can become objective as you eat. Of course, as long as you are guilty of the sin of pride, you will not be able to become truly objective, to your eating or to anything else. You will be eating to escape reality and to build up your ego and, also, to escape the guilt of doing so. However, if you can let go of enough egotism and pride to get beyond the fear of dying, you will be able to catch glimpses of my meaning.

You came into the world in a relatively pure state, but a combination of food and emotionality soon caused you to evolve a dual nature: the inwardly related nature, the "you" of your birth (the real you), and the outwardly related animal nature (the "not-you") that is so dear to our decadent society.

It was this latter nature your mother unwittingly served as she rocked your cradle and prepared your food, passing along as she did so, from her generation to yours, the food-addicted, death-oriented spores of pride to sustain your sibling (not-you) nature. As a result, the real you didn't grow up at all—*it* (the not-you) did. And have you noticed how the more you feed a hungry ego, the hungrier it gets? It can never be satisfied.

In my writings I have endeavored to show by examining and exposing your current habits how the human race descended via a food/woman-based rebellion against the ultimate authority (God) to the egocentric, sensual way of life we are now caught up in. Glorifying the present man/woman arrangement is the pervasive serpent-based system of culture we call civilization, headed by female-imprinted male leaders, deceivers, and liars to the core. Young people love to hate these authorities with whom they are hopelessly caught up in a deadly pattern of rebellion and conformity.

Descended man craves worldly love; descended woman has learned to crave a falling man's passion for her. He needs the emotional excitement awakened by her lie love, and she lives on the miasma of his emotional decay. A woman evolves her female nature as she falls into a dependency on a man's weakness, and she soon becomes addicted to her feelings of contempt for him. As he sets her up to be an object of use to support his ego, she is compelled in self-defense to set him up to fail through the lying love he demands of her. A man can always be counted on to fall for food and sex, and he falls to sex through food. As he indulges his craving for food and sex, it doesn't take long for him to develop other contemptible weaknesses.

Mankind is being killed by food poisoning, and men are dying from a malignant relationship with women. Women die alone on this wretched earth, having unwittingly, with less reason than the black widow spider, killed their mates. And what is more, it is the way women (who since time immemorial have been tutored in the sexy culinary arts) prepare the spicy concoctions that causes the mutual downfall of woman and man. This domestic relationship has its counterpart in the larger world where powerful authorities get elected into the power elite in the same way that men elect their women goddesses. Thus, all men get the kind of government (and the kind of women) they richly deserve.

Women use cultural culinary skills to "keep the

family together" and keep them under the spell of the ages. The woman is the cultural seat of power. Her food bonds man's will to hers. God forgive her, for she can't realize that her will is not her own, but is subject to the spirit of Original Sin, and thus, the food she offers to please her man is the downfall of them both. He has always fallen through her food and sex, and she has fallen from grace and love through being tempted to hate his weakness for her.

This is a very important point to remember: Through Original Sin, man has metamorphosed to take on the spirit of the female identity. The first spiritual man became sensual man. Notice how every time you do a forbidden thing—indulge in a forbidden thought, perhaps—you become more sensual and less of a person; grosser animal feelings and desires spring up in you, along with a fear of impending death.

To serve any soul guilefully is to rule it. To feed an ego with lies and food and sex is to create obligation, obedience, and allegiance—all kinds of longings and weaknesses that need soothing and servicing. Through food, perhaps more than through any of her other ministrations, a woman is enabled to commit the perfect crime. *Serving* seems so innocent that it is never suspected for what it is. Indeed, *any* gift offering can create a powerful obligation, even if it is just a "free" flower at the airport in exchange for a donation. Under the circumstances, the victim cannot refuse the hidden demand to part with a portion of his soul along with his money. The taker is taken.

A delicious fresh apple attests to the glory of God; but who is honored when it is cooked down into a tempting plate of apple strudel? Surely, glory goes to the chef. From this food service, a woman develops an irresistible compulsion to serve and please the source of that glory, the prideful fool who falls for her love offering. A very subtle principle is contained here. It encompasses the entire spectrum of manipulative giving, all the way down to such an *apparently* charitable thing as welfare.

Because ego reinforcement from the mother spirit is basic to our perverse need, we go for the strudel rather than a nice fresh apple from the table of God. Corrupted food is ego-comforting food, more attractive and appealing than what is truly natural and good. Your ego is threatened, and you feel cheated whenever you are deprived of your regular fix: some hot, steamy, delectable cultural concoction. For what we are all really seeking in our piggy slop is the familiar reinforcing spirit of the ambitious, rebellious, fallen state of mind.

How difficult it is for us to realize that we are cheating ourselves of God's Salvation by our mindless indulgences, but we must one day wake up to the fact that we are feeding the dark side of our nature with every bite. Our altered need is so great that we cannot separate feeding our ego from satisfying normal body needs.

So, as we feed our egos, we tend to poison our real selves. Forgive the redundancy, but I must remind you that every time we eat anything, even good, natural food, we are reinforcing the alien self.

This is especially true in the case of food you do not earn, food eaten in anger, and even health food if you are eating it as a way to salvation or to cure your diseases.

Ideally, you should eat sensibly, for doing so has some value, but that practice alone cannot save your soul. Eating properly may lead to better health, but even then you dare not eat with the motive of salvation. Such motivation converts your eating habits into yet another ego trip to damn you. Good food alone has no power to save you from the sentence you are serving for having eaten forbidden food. You must beware of that sort of deception.

Ever since the Fall of man, men have had problems with food through women. The curse projected through women awakened sexual desires leading to woman/food abuse and causing them to become so fixated on women that women have become a god to men, a ground of their being.

Everything an ambitious man does is for female approval. His mind dwells on her continuously as though she were his god. She becomes powerful in her contemptuous servicing of his weakness, a weakness that she knows will be the death of her but that she must continue to serve if she is to have any man/woman relationship at all.

A really hateful female conceals her pleasure in judgment behind an offering of food. The madder she gets at her husband, the more she enjoys "fixing" him through his belly. So, through food and sex, a woman "loves"—and gets her revenge. The stupid fool is so eager to fall, to use, to gratify his piggy self, that as he bellies up to her table, she bellies up to him to feed her judgment and to live off his dying to her. She derives an ugly satisfaction out of reducing him to a grunting pig.

Men and women both take great pleasure in degrading one another, evolving each other's ego animals as tyrant gods and slaves in a living hell. Some forms of overweight are caused by frustration of a woman feeding a male identity in herself. Conversely, some men have a woman inside them preparing their meals; they just love food and love to cook.

Food is charged with dream value, and fantasy is the stuff of which pride is made. No matter how you slice it, food—especially the junk stuff—has a hypnotic power to dull the mind and reinforce identity, dependency, wimpishness, and later, rebellious and violent animal behavior. Either way—the way of the wimp or the way of the beast—hell's purpose is served.

Allegiance to false gods is intensified through the ritual of eating. We all eat to "remember" who and what we are. That remembering also has a forgetting side that allows us to exist in a trancelike state for as long as we are involved with a feeling self aroused by food poison. It is a form of somnambulism. Throughout our lives, we eat and sleepwalk in an eerie reverie. As an example, there is a popular restaurant in California that takes its name from the Greek word for *a potion used to induce forgetfulness of pain or sorrow* and offers delicious food and spectacular views to enhance the sensuous, hypnotic dining experience.

We eat to forget, but make no mistake about it; our minds will not be empty. Forgetting has its remembering side. And a crafty woman never lets a man forget that he is a man. Without her constant reminders, he might remember the truth that he is not a man and become anxious and conscience-stricken. Man lives in hell with woman, though he may think it is heaven. Without her, he sees the truth that he is in hell. And how does he get back into heaven's grace? Why, through a sex and eating binge!

The delusion produced by food and sex is almost flawless. With our fix we think we are gods in heaven. Without the fix, we see that we are slaves in hell, but we imagine that our plight is due to our not being loyal enough to the source of our ego pleasure and fulfillment. The same idea comes to mind as we try to break away from drink, drugs, or a relationship—even with church.

Ritualistic cultural food is a magic potion that makes you forget you are falling by feeding you the illusion that you are a beautiful being gloriously rising. To go on believing in this delusion, you must be fed a steady diet of cultural, ritualistic ego food. Then you "awaken" in this dream we all share, as a god, in the same state Alice was in on the other side of the looking glass—that is, she simply didn't know that she was asleep.

The very idea of giving up ritualistic food and sex, which are supportive of our egocentric lifestyle, along with music and all sorts of mind-altering addictions, makes us feel as though we'd be opening the door to death and hell, forsaking life, duty, and all the things that make life bearable on earth. You see, don't you, how stubbornly we cling to the illusion of our dream state that we are awake and living as gods and masters of our fate? And how a true awakening could be a death threat to the "glorious" life of the sense-based alien self?

We are, for the most part, living life with a back-to-front perspective on reality that has been part and parcel of our thought stuff ever since the culture of our environment projected us into this altered state of consciousness.

Most of us, like those Japanese kamikaze pilots, would rather go to "heaven," commit hara-kiri with our Jim Joneses, psychopaths, alcohol, drugs, and Twinkies, though it be the death of us, than lose face and wake up and see what fools we are. That is why the system killed, and still kills, iconoclasts like Socrates, Jesus Christ, and anyone else graced with true nobility.

We are all born subject to wicked and powerful teachers, leaders, and priests, whom our parents in their madness elected to stroke their egos. Our parents have laid us on the altar of these authorities like sacrificial lambs, to be brainwashed by a process they call "education." We grow up in a society where evil deception is king, where innocence is degraded and crucified.

The false gods that have risen to power through the weaknesses of the generations that preceded us are very jealous gods indeed. They are also dangerous. Ruthless with those they perceive to be a threat to their system, they will not let unlettered iconoclastic challengers rise to question their authority. Aware, self-controlled, thoughtful children who reserve the right to look before they leap are seen as misfits or troublemakers.

The average fool falls right in with the system, and the innocent are thrown to the lions. The favored fool, who is actually being fattened for the kill, never lets a second of space exist between delights. Nor would the devil permit it. Were the truth all around him, watching for a tiny bit of space through which to shine upon his soul, truth's vigil would be in vain. Our average fool would be too inebriated, too bewitched by the indulgences he looks on as the good life to know it was there.

He is too busy titillating his ego. While enjoying a steak, he looks forward to dessert; over dessert, he looks forward to his after-dinner drink; while drinking, he lustily anticipates the pleasure of his next sexual encounter. The stubborn fool goes on rejecting the Salvation of God by clinging to his ego life through his trauma-based piggish pleasures.

Idolators, worshipers at shrines made in the image of their own selfishness, are deathly afraid of the light that shines in honest men and women. The masses fear real live teachers, preferring professional death-centered liars who have themselves been sacrificed on the altars of culture. The stupid masses enjoy being degraded by sociopaths. Why? When the black light of corruption turns its spotlight on them, their animal is aroused, and their souls feel like those of gods coming into existence; each beast thinks that it is a god man.

Behold the churches, politicians, "healing arts" motivators and manipulators, exploiters of all kinds. These are the architects of our death-centered culture.

Ancient wise men fasted and prayed because they knew that all food clouds the reason, shielding it from its original nutrient light. But the only antidote to the food sin is, first, repentance and then the Eucharist. Catholic theologians call a soul's defection from the satanic system to the will of God the *Eucharist* (from the French and Greek words meaning "to favor or give grace to a spiritual yearning"). The only ritual Christ left behind for his followers involved their eating of bread, symbolic of his flesh, and drinking the wine, symbolic of his spirit, in remembrance of him.

During your next meal, observe (if you can) how food affects your mind. The hypnosis of the first bite is so instantaneous and complete that *you* disappear. You are suddenly and mysteriously less aware, and you have probably never been conscious of the fact that this has happened to you. It is a very difficult thing to observe, because the drug-like effect is so traumatically and posthypnotically implanted and so uplifting that even if you do try to catch yourself dreaming (escaping), you may not succeed. It is like trying to catch yourself falling asleep. You can stay conscious just so long, and then the sleep (sin) state bewitches you; you forget to remember. You may get as far as to sit down at the table with the idea of remembering to eat in His memory, but with the first bite you are lost in food-induced thought. *This is because no one can eat of the body of Christ's redemption until he has repented of his selfish life.*

You see, I hope, what the problem is: food causes instant daydreaming, instant forgetfulness, comfort, escape. Flowing up through the food experience comes the flesh-and-spirit reinforcement of our fallen identity. Food poisons our relationship with God through its appeal to the *not-you* self that is dependent on the poisoning spirit of food. You feed your ego, and your body becomes mean, old, and ugly—barely recognizable as the *you* of your youth.

Food not only poisons your relationship with God and deadens the soul, but it also poisons the body as its evil spirit works its way in. Perfectly honorable men live and die without ever discovering the mystery of the food sin. Food is the last piece of the puzzle of Salvation, coming, as it does, after we have been made aware and have repented of the many sensual hang-ups of the past that evolved from the poisoned apple. Food is loaded with terrible dream suggestions. Food makes us guilty, and food makes us "innocent" again. We are addicted to food for the security of false innocence; food is full of lies, disease, and death.

Now Christ has intercepted Satan's suggestion that death is life, and He has done so through food. Great wisdom is needed here. Behold a mystery: whosoever is graced to recognize the Christ as the Son of God, our Redeemer, and who can by grace repent of pride, forbear to hate, use, and blame others and can prove a commitment to God by his actions, can receive the "body" of Christ.

The Last Supper is, without doubt, Original Sin revisited and undone. Through the forbidden fruit, man identified with the spirit of evil. He took on its mortal physical form and spiritual purpose. Christ reverses the purpose of hell on earth and frees us from bondage to it when he commands us to eat his body (bread) and drink his blood (wine).

Through faith, the hell-bound personality that has been looking to food for its justified life becomes divinely transformed. We evolve a new creature, remolded through our mind from within. This new creature translates the will of God through the Holy Spirit, and his entire being is transformed through all the persecution he must suffer.

The Evil One, working through woman and food, lied when he said that the fruit could awaken man to the knowledge that he could be God. To this day, we rebel against the supreme authority and fantasize ourselves to be great through food's reinforcing power.

But through His only begotten son, God has reconciled us to himself. God has changed the effect food has on us, once and for all. The same food may, by command of hell's immortal enemy, become charged with a different force. Food partaken of in mindfulness of Him becomes an antidote to the order of the serpent that has come down to us through the word of women. The Holy Spirit, acting now through a man/food principle, countermands the order of the food/female principality. Do you see it?

The Eucharist of the Church is not the real thing. The body of Christ is not a wafer, holy or otherwise. Christ is, however, in every bite that is truly eaten in remembrance of him until he comes again—and this, only for those who truly love God.

Therefore, whosoever eats the bread and drinks the cup of the Lord in an unworthy manner (i.e., phony, plastic show of ritual) *will be guilty of sinning against the body and blood of the Lord. For anyone who eats and drinks without recognizing the body of the Lord, drinks judgment on himself.*

—I Corinthians 11:27, 29

Also:

That is why so many among you are weak and sick and many have fallen asleep (died). *We are being disciplined so we'll not be condemned with the world.*

—I Corinthians 11:30, 32

This cup is the new testament in my blood. This do ye as oft as ye drink it in remembrance of me.

—I Corinthians 11:25

The word *Eucharist* is similar in meaning to the word *charisma*—literally "the good gift of favor or grace, beatific personality."

This blessed (from the old English *blithe*, as in "blithe spirit"), carefree personality is formed by the inbreathing of the new indwelling spirit. In the Christ's Salvation, you have new life, breathed in through a new belief system. Food eaten while mindful of his sacrifice and his new order changes you from within. You come under the command of God, through his obedient son and his true word, the spirit of truth handed down through man as opposed to the lying spirit that came up through women. The old order of sin was Satan's will in women to put woman's nature in man, whereby man unwittingly takes the supporting role in the drama of hell on earth.

So the way you relate to food profoundly changes the way you relate as a man to all women. And the woman who prepares the food simply, not putting too much of herself into its preparation (in order to seduce her man into adoring her) is blessed by partaking of the Lord of her husband, who, provided he requires nothing fancier of her, is blessed of the Christ.

Remember, through the fruit of disobedience, man took on the woman's spirit and the woman's identity. Now, through the Lord's Supper, we take on the spirit of truth (the wine) and his flesh, his body, through the bread. That is the meaning of "eating his flesh and drinking his blood," for it is from this that we take on his identity and become a new creature.

Most of us are the sum total of our experiences, but another way of saying this is that we are burdened down and bothered by our past. Unless we learn to respond properly in the present moment, the present becomes merely an extension of that burdensome past.

Roy Masters, author of this persuasive self-help book, describes a remarkably simple technique to help us face life properly, calmly. He shows us that it is the way we respond emotionally to pressures that makes us sick and depressed.

By leading us back to our center of dignity and understanding and showing us how to apply one simple principle, Roy Masters shows us how to remain sane, poised and tranquil under the most severe trials and tribulations.

Roy Masters has nothing less to offer you than the secret of life itself—how to get close to yourself and find your lost identity, the true self you have lost in the confusion.

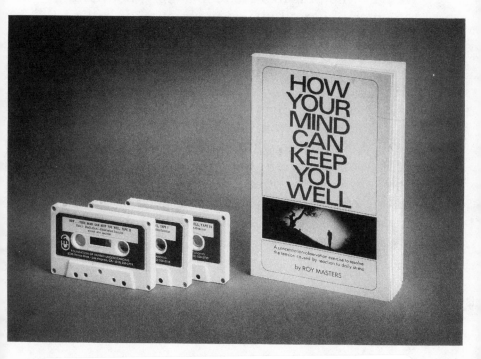

Other Books Available

The Foundation of Human Understanding
P.O. Box 1009 - Grants Pass - OR - 97528

HOW TO CONTROL YOUR EMOTIONS
Simple instructions by which anyone may learn how to eliminate guilt, anxiety, pain, and suffering from his life forever, completely and without effort. 325 pages

HOW TO CONQUER SUFFERING WITHOUT DOCTORS
The relationship that now exists between you and your healer is the relationship which should exist within yourself. This book shows the seeker how to look inside himself for common sense and answers that are meaningful and permanent. 222 pages

SEX, SIN & SALVATION
This work explains how man's failing ego expresses itself in terms of sex and violence and how husband and wife can eventually transcend their sexual problems. 321 pages

SECRET OF LIFE
A philosophical guide to the whole riddle of existence. 194 pages

NO ONE HAS TO DIE!
There lives in this world an insidious evil force that understands and caters to our weakness, and we are delivered into the hands of the evil shepherd, and he is the author of our suffering or tragedy until we find the truth that makes us free. 243 pages

THE SATAN PRINCIPLE
The entire thrust of this book is to bring all the subtle causes of your problems into the spotlight of your consciousness. 261 pages

HEALERS, GURUS, AND SPIRITUAL GUIDES
ESP, psychic healing and mind-over-matter explained in this easy-to-read book by William Wolff. Several chapters are devoted to Roy Masters, informative biographical material plus case histories of meditation at work. 258 pages

HOW TO SURVIVE YOUR PARENTS
Since all parents were once children, the question arises: How can we survive our parents; how do our children survive us? In no uncertain terms, this book tells how. 190 pages

THE ADAM & EVE *SINDROME*
In our present state, we can hardly have a relationship that isn't wrong. It is imperative, Masters says, to see directly to the original cause with objective precision . . . and then, in that moment of realization, the curse is broken. 266 pages

EAT NO EVIL
The ultimate book on food—a delightfully shocking expose' of what is at the very root of all your food hang-ups. 157 pages

* OUR PRICES HAVE CHANGED *
Please contact us for a complete catalog

Suggested Materials

INTRODUCTION TO MATERIALS

The Foundation of Human Understanding was founded by Roy Masters in 1961. With a listening audience of over one million, The Foundation of Human Understanding has gained worldwide prominence and recognition in the field of helping people understand and solve personal and family problems. Roy Masters' syndicated radio program, "How Your Mind Can Keep You Well," can now be heard throughout the entire United States, Canada, portions of Central America, and ten European countries.

To date, The Foundation of Human Understanding estimates having sold over 350,000 books written by Roy Masters, and an equal number of cassette tapes of Masters' radio call-in program, and various lectures and recorded seminars. These figures may not be initially all that impressive, but bear in mind that for twenty-four years Masters has been hosting his live one-hour call-in program from Los Angeles, California, literally giving away the answers to questions and problems in such a precise manner, that most callers and listeners alike glean what they need in just a few moments.

Roy Masters is not in his line of work for profit. He loves what he does; but most of all, he loves people. Here are a few quotes from his daily radio show: "What I enjoy doing most is waking people up from their hypnotic trances." "If I love you, then I see to it that you need me less." "If you have true love, you will not identify with another person, nor will you allow anyone you love to identify with you."

The subjects listed below are loaded with insightful answers to almost any question you have. These materials are only available through The Foundation of Human Understanding.

OBSERVATION PACKAGE

In order to gain control over thoughts and feelings, you must learn to become objective, to separate from your subjective thought stream. The observation exercise helps you regain the ability to focus your attention, thus returning you to self-discipline and the power of concentration.

"How Your Mind Can Keep You Well"

Instruction in the basic technique of observation as taught by Roy Masters. Consists of three compact cassettes and a book by the same name. $30

The basic observation technique is also available in Spanish. Please refer to tape number 4588 when ordering. $10 per 90 min. cassette tape.

If you cannot afford the price of the observation materials, it is the policy of the Foundation to allow you to pay what you can afford. Please be fair.

BOOKS

In each of Roy Masters' books, he zeros in on the specific causes and effects that emotions play in our personal behavior and social life and offers positive answers and insights that will change the way you react to the pressure and strain of everyday life.

1. How Your Mind Can Keep You Well
2. How to Control Your Emotions
3. How to Conquer Suffering Without Doctors
4. The Secret of Life
5. Sex, Sin & Salvation
6. No One Has to Die
7. The Satan Principle
8. Healers, Gurus & Spiritual Guides (by William Wolff)

THE SIX PACK

"How to Control Your Emotions Through Observation"

These six compact cassette tapes contain an expanded discussion of the Basic Observation Exercise and the principles which are revealed through its practice. The cost is $36 per set, and an additional $4 for a handy binder (optional).

1. The Truth About One's Nothingness—Resentment *(#1004)*
2. Release from Thoughts—Awareness of Hypnosis *(#1005)*
3. Finding Your Conscience—Freedom from Gurus *(#1006)*
4. Worry—Meditation is Awareness *(#1007)*
5. Resentment—Responding to Children *(#1008)*
6. Doubt, Fear, & Faith *(#1009)*

NEW DIMENSIONS

New Dimensions is a magazine dedicated to helping you understand and deal with the problems and pressures of everyday life. Each issue of *New Dimensions* presents eye-opening insights into familiar and often difficult personal and family problems such as: sex, love, anxiety, bad habits, disease, and death. *New Dimensions* leaves no subject untouched, attempting to expose and dispel the misconceptions that plague our modern society. Perhaps the most accurate description of this fast-growing publication would be: a mind-expanding resource of insights, new ideas, and spiritually uplifting information that stimulates higher thinking and positive action.

You will receive 12 monthly issues, each containing information and articles that could change your life and save you thousands of dollars by providing you with provocative answers to problems doctors and psychiatrists haven't even begun to understand.

To subscribe to *New Dimensions* write to: The Foundation of Human Understanding, P.O. Box 34036, Los Angeles, CA 90034, or P.O. Box 811, Grants Pass, OR 97526.

Subscription rates:

U.S.: one year $36 third class; two years $66. One year $48 first class; two years $90. Foreign: one year $52 surface; two years $98. One year $78 A.O. Air; two years $150.

TAPE OF THE MONTH

Every month we put together the most intriguing conversations between Roy Masters and callers, and call it "The Tape of the Month." Each 90-minute cassette is edited from over forty hours of live radio, to showcase the most interesting and enlightening segments of each month's broadcasts.

You can receive a full year's subscription (12 cassettes) by sending $100 for third class; $112 for first class; $140 overseas air, or you may order individual tapes by sending $10 plus $1.00 postage and handling ($1.75 first class or UPS), and identify the tape you want by month and year. Address your orders to: "Tape-of-the-Month Club," c/o The Foundation of Human Understanding.

VIDEOTAPES

Please specify Beta or VHS format and remember to add $5 for UPS shipping and handling, and $6 for overseas delivery.

Now you can experience the powerful awakening of Roy Masters' lectures and seminars in the comfort and privacy of your home. Videotapes give you the time to absorb the message and meaning at your own speed and without the usual interruptions and delays involved with attending a large gathering, and are a good way to introduce your friends and family to the way of Roy Masters.

Tape #1 The Quest for Life
The Ventura Healing Seminar

This ten-hour program is the most in-depth of the four tapes and contains a detailed discussion of all facets of hate. Also included is a thorough demonstration on how to stop smoking where Roy uses the cross on several people from the audience. This is a very unique tape. The cost is $175.

Tape #2 The Hypnosis/Healing Seminar, Los Angeles Marriott Hotel

This five-hour program contains actual exorcisms and onstage healings, and in-depth discussions on the hypnosis of life. The cost is $100.

Tape #3 Finding the Light Within
Dealing With Problems & Pressures Through Observation

This two-hour program is a good introductory tape dealing with the basic principles of understanding pressure, and correct practice of meditation. Also included is a 20-minute documentary about Tall Timber Ranch in Oregon. Good for family and friends. The cost is $35.

THE PROGRAM

Listening to the program, "How Your Mind Can Keep You Well" on the radio with Roy Masters as host to troubled callers can be a very enlightening experience, because we can all identify with a particular caller's problem and somehow magically glean valuable insights into our own.

For only $6 plus the cost of postage and handling, you can purchase individual radio program tapes by identifying the tape you want by program number. Address your orders to: The Foundation of Human Understanding, P.O. Box 34036, Los Angeles, CA 90034.

TELEVISED VIDEOTAPES

Please specify Beta or VHS format and remember to add $5 for UPS shipping and handling, and $6 for overseas delivery.

Thanks to modern video technology, you can now "attend" some of Roy Masters' best lectures and seminars without leaving your living room. The following list of videotapes are actual discussion groups with audience participation that have been given by Roy Masters at The Foundation of Human Understanding in Los Angeles, California, and are later aired over various television stations on the west coast. Now you can purchase these videotapes to view in

the privacy of your own home, should his television program not yet be available in your particular area. They are also a great way to introduce friends and family to The Foundation of Human Understanding. Note: The majority of these lectures are also available on audio cassette. See Suggested Materials List for prices.

Overcoming Family Problems (#4429) 120 min./$35

Learning to Overcome Compulsive Habits (#4443) 120 min./$35

Sexual Conflict: The Cause & Cure (#4453) 120 min./$35

Mind Over Malady (#4463) 120 min./$35

Marriage & Divorce: The Cause & Cure (#4473) 60 min./$25

The Crisis of Faith Through Emotions (#4492) 60 min./$25

Reversing the Process of Old Age (#4483) 120 min./$35

Masters, MacKenzie, & Antonio "AIDS Cover-Up" Special (#4479) 60 min./$25

The Mechanics of Meditation (#4482) 60 min./$25

Overcoming Self Doubt (#4493) 150 min./$50

Trauma: Past & Present (#4503) 150 min./$50

The Alien Identity Within (#4509) 150 min./$50

How to Survive Your Mother & Wife (#4511) 150 min./$50

LECTURES ON . . .

Roy Masters has been lecturing for 25 years on topics ranging from Finding God to Psychic Vampirism. There is literally no subject concerning human emotions that he has left unexamined.

MEDITATION

Basics of Meditation (#1160) 90 min./$10

The Key to Meditation (#1961) 90 min./$10

Advanced Techniques of Meditation (#1176) 90 min./$10

Is Meditation for Christians? (#1944 1 & 2) 120 min./$12

Exploring the Meditative Life (#4337) 90 min./$10

The Mechanics of Meditation (#4482) 60 min./$10

ROY MASTERS SPEAKS

In this special series, specific subjects are selected from Roy Masters' daily radio broadcasts and compiled onto a 90-minute (unless otherwise specified) cassette tape.

Man-Woman Relations, Part 1 (#1371) 60 min./$10
Man-Woman Relations, Part 2 (#1786) 90 min./$10
Man-Woman Relations, Part 3 (#1840) 90 min./$10
Man-Woman Relations, Part 4 (#2615) 90 min./$10
Man-Woman Relations, Part 5 (#2807) 90 min./$10
Man-Woman Relations, Part 6 (#4187) 90 min./$10
Man-Woman Relations, Part 7 (#4373) 90 min./$10
Man-Woman Relations, Part 8 (#4439) 90 min./$10
Resolving Family Problems (#1388) 90 min./$10
The Power of Words (#1399) 90 min./$10
Why Children Have Problems (#1410) 90 min./$10
Injustice (#1413) 90 min./$10
Dealing Properly With Children (#1441) 90 min./$10
The Effects of Music (#1525) 90 min./$10
The Meaning of Faith (#1599) 90 min./$10
False Belief (#1605) 90 min./$10
The Power of Realization (#1608) 90 min./$10
Understanding the Lower Self (#1699) 90 min./$10
Pride, the Cause of Death (#1750) 90 min./$10
All About Judgment (#2351) 90 min./$10
So You Don't Think There's a Devil, Eh? (#2423) 65 min./$10
Homosexuality: The Cause (#2443) 90 min./$10
Overcoming Overeating (#2464) 90 min./$10
Tyrants & Wimps (#2596) 90 min./$10
Willfulness (#2665) 90 min./$10
Understanding Failure: The Key to Success (#2699) 90 min.$10
Confusing Women, Confounded Men (#2719) 90 min./$10
Friends, Family & Speaking Up (#2737) 90 min./$10
Vanity (#2817) 90 min./$10
Doubt, Insecurity and Starting Your Own Business (#2903) 90 min./$10
Guiding Children With Common Sense (#2947) 90 min./$10
How to Give Up Smoking (#2991) 90 min./$10
Male Sexuality (#2993 1 & 2) 180 min./$20
Female Sexuality (#2995 1 & 2) 180 min./$20
Diseases of Resentment (#3083 1 & 2) 180 min./$20

Roy Masters Talks to Kids (#4169) 90 min./$10
Learning to Live Without Worry (#4297) 90 min./$10

HEALTH

Healing (#1682) 90 min./$10
Faith Healing (#2030 1 & 2) 130 min./$12
Faith & Hope (#1875) 90 min./$10
Sickness & Disease (#1220) 90 min./$10
Cancer & Heart Attacks (#1602) 90 min./$10
Death & Dying—Life & Living (#1112-1113) 120 min./$12
Alcoholism: The Cause and Cure (#2575) 60 min./$10
Food, Damnation & Salvation (#2835 1 & 2) 180 min./$20
Reversing the Process of Old Age (#4483) 120 min./$12

RELIGION

Finding God (#2140) 60 min./$10
Be Still & Know (#1601 1 & 2) 120 min./$12
Beyond Knowlege (#1510 1 & 2) 180 min./$20
Secret Path to the Paradise State (#1116 1 & 2) 120 min./$12
Creation vs. Evolution (#2252) 90 min./$10
Overcoming Evil (#2256) 90 min./$10
What it Really Means to Conquer Evil (#2452) 90 min./$10
The Crisis of Faith & Doubt (#2633) 90 min./$10
Antidote to Original Sin (#3053) 90 min./$10
How Evil Begins and Ends (#3065 1 & 2) 120 min./$12
The Sins of the Fathers (#4021) 90 min./$10
Finding the Teacher Within (#4271) 90 min./$10
What it Really Means to be Born Again (#4465) 90 min./$10
The Mystical Meaning of Christmas (#4523) 120 min./$12

SUCCESS & SURVIVAL

How to Survive Your Mother and Wife (#4511) 150 min./$20

Masters, McKenzie, & Antonio
"The AIDS Cover-Up" Special (#4479) 60 min./$6

Politicians and the AIDS Virus: Can
America Survive Them? (#4472) 90 min./$10

The Principles of Success
(#4421) Mark Masters 120 min./$12

Investing and Relocating in Oregon
(#4433) Mark Masters 120 min./$12

How to Win an Argument (#4357) 90 min./$10

How to Solve All Your Problems
(#4234) 140 min./$16

Violence in the Family and Nation
(#4270) 90 min./$10

What is Destroying America (#4088) 90 min./$10

How to Survive in a Society Gone Crazy
(#4029) 90 min./$10

Moral & Financial Survival (#2131) 60 min./$10

Success Without Ambition (#1921) 90 min./$10

Success Without Destruction (#1922) 90 min./$10

Success Without Guilt (#4321) 90 min./$10

SPECIAL SEMINARS

Hypnosis of Life—Oregon '81
(#1905 1 & 2) 180 min./$20

Hypnosis of Life—Boston '84
(#2853 1, 2, 3, & 4) 360 min./$36

Hypnosis of Life—San Francisco '85
(#2948 1, 2, 3, & 4) 360 min./$36

Hypnosis of Life—San Francisco '87
(#4425 1 & 2) 180 min./$20

EMOTIONAL PROBLEMS

Understanding Emotions (#1240) 90 min./$10

Emotional Blocks (#1888) 90 min./$10

The Secrets of Dealing With Stress
(#2196) 90 min./$10

Happiness (#1883) 90 min./$10

Bad Habits (#1375) 90 min./$10

Psychic Vampirism (#1705) 90 min./$10

The Truth About Sex (#2112) 90 min./$10

Sex & Violence—Love & Hate (#1188) 90 min./$10

Addiction to Drugs, Sex & Alcohol
(#1962) 90 min./$10

The Dangers of Music
(#2195) David Masters 90 min./$10

Dominance & Subservience (#2048) 60 min./$10

Identity—Uncovering the True Self
(#1960) 90 min./$10

Conquering the Suggestive Power of Words
(#1500 1 & 2) 180 min./$20

Secrets of Salvation (#1270) 90 min./$10

Marriage: It Doesn't Have to Be a Living Hell
(#2315) 90 min./$10

Bigotry (#2369) 90 min./$10

Selfishness (#2397) 90 min./$10

Change Your Attitude—Change Your Destiny
(#2629 1 & 2) 120 min./$12

Dealing With Wicked Authority
(#2631) 90 min./$10

A Deeper Look Into Family Problems
(#2557) 90 min./$10

Becoming Perfect (#2767) 90 min./$10

The Blessings and Benefits of a Poor Memory
(#2822) 90 min./$10

Revenge and Forgiveness (#2823) 120 min./$12

You Don't Have to Be Ruled by Inferior Beings
(#2929) 90 min./$10

Resolving Past Sins (#2939) 90 min./$10

Seeking the Blessed State of Mind
(#2975) 90 min./$10

Forgiveness (#3069) 90 min./$10

Understanding the Subconscious Mind
(#4381) 90 min./$10

Happiness or Misery (#4423) 90 min./$10

Understanding vs. Knowledge (#4435) 90 min./$10

Learning to Overcome Compulsive Habits
(#4443) 120 min./$12

Sexual Conflict: The Cause & Cure
(#4453) 120 min./$12

Mind Over Malady (#4463) 120 min./$12

Marriage & Divorce: The Cause & Cure
(#4473) 60 min./$10

The Crisis of Faith Through Emotions
(#4492) 60 min./$10

Breaking Free From Addictions
(#4331) 90 min./$10

Dealing Correctly With Stress (#4338) 90 min./$10

Overcoming Self Doubt (#4493) 150 min./$20

Trauma: Past & Present (#4503) 150 min./$20

The Alien Identity Within (#4509) 150 min./$20